THE *Skinny*
15 MINUTE MEALS
& *YOGA* WORKOUT PLAN

CookNation

THE SKINNY 15 MINUTE MEALS & YOGA WORKOUT PLAN
CALORIE COUNTED 15 MINUTE MEALS WITH GENTLE YOGA WORKOUTS FOR HEALTH & WELLBEING

ISBN 978-1-911219-50-7

A CIP catalogue record of this book is available from the British Library

• •

DISCLAIMER

Some recipes may contain nuts or traces of nuts. Those suffering from any allergies associated with nuts should avoid any recipes containing nuts or nut based oils.
This information is provided and sold with the knowledge that the publisher and author do not offer any legal or other professional advice.
In the case of a need for any such expertise consult with the appropriate professional.
This book does not contain all information available on the subject, and other sources of recipes are available.

A basic level of fitness is required to perform the workouts in this book. Any health concerns should be discussed with a health professional before embarking on any of the exercises detailed.

This book has not been created to be specific to any individual's requirements. Every effort has been made to make this book as accurate as possible. However, there may be typographical and or content errors. Therefore, this book should serve only as a general guide and not as the ultimate source of subject information.

This book contains information that might be dated and is intended only to educate and entertain.

The author and publisher shall have no liability or responsibility to any person or entity regarding any loss or damage incurred, or alleged to have incurred, directly or indirectly, by the information contained in this book.

CONTENTS

DINNER

INTRODUCTION

If you are time-poor but want to eat healthy, delicious, nutritious meals every day AND boost your physical & mental wellbeing....you can, and all in 15 minutes or less!

In our fast paced way of life, healthy, balanced and nutritious meals are often the first thing to be compromised. "I haven't got time to cook", "I'll eat on the go" or "I'll skip lunch and eat later" are just some of the excuses we all use throughout our hectic lives resulting in poor diet choices, sluggishness and weight gain.

If you are following a diet, meal choices, as well as daily exercise can become even more difficult and the added pressure of finding time to prepare food can cause you to fall at the first hurdle.

Here's the good news. If you are time-poor but want to eat healthy, delicious and nutritious meals every day AND boost your physical and mental wellbeing through yoga... you can, and all in 15 minutes or less! **The Skinny 15 Minute Meals & Yoga Workout Plan** brings over 60 breakfast, lunch and dinner recipes to the table in 15 minutes or less and all below 300, 400 or 500 calories each. Plus our gentle yoga workouts are fully illustrated with simple instructions to perform at home .

If you think you haven't got time to cook and exercise...think again. You could be eating delicious, skinny, fat burning meals and gentle yoga routines every day in just 15 minutes.

The majority of recipes serve one and are big on flavour and nutrition – no compromises.

THE SECRET TO 15 MINUTE MEALS

Preparing and cooking meals in 15 minutes or less requires a little help from modern convenience stores in the shape of some carefully selected pre-prepared products. Slashing prep times is how you can make 15 minutes meals in a flash.

By altering your shopping habits a little, your fridge and store cupboard can be regularly stocked with super-fast pre-prepared ingredients that make meals simple – less time, less fuss, less washing up! We're not talking highly processed fast food but instead, freshly prepared ingredients that will save you the time chopping, washing, peeling, grating and all the other laborious tasks that add minutes to your kitchen prep.

To follow is a list of some of the most common pre-prepared smart buys used in our recipes that will slash time off your cooking. This is not however a comprehensive shopping list, so check which recipes you plan to follow and shop accordingly.

- Jar crushed chilli flakes
- Bags pre sliced/chopped onions
- Bags pre sliced/chopped red onions
- Bags prepared carrot batons
- Bags washed, sliced mushrooms
- Bags washed rocket, spinach and mixed salad leaves
- Bags prepared shredded kale & spring greens
- Packets trimmed asparagus tips
- Packets trimmed green beans
- Packets shelled fresh peas
- Pre-grated low fat cheddar cheese
- Pre-grated Parmesan cheese
- Packets straight-to-wok noodles
- Packets ready-to-go microwaveable rice
- Bottle of lime juice
- Bottle of lemon juice
- Jar sundried tomatoes in oil
- Curry powder
- Pre-cooked chicken breasts

Remember that pre-prepared just means someone has already done some of the work for you. The ingredients we suggest are still nutritious, fresh and full of flavour – no compromises on taste or goodness. Adding these items may add a few extra pennies to your weekly shopping budget but the time you'll save in the kitchen will be worth it. Plus you'll be eating great-tasting, healthy, calorie counted meals every day…in just 15 minutes.

You could of course prepare many of these ingredients yourself when you have more time and have them ready in the fridge to use when preparing your 15 minute meals.

PREPARATION & COOKING TIMES

All the recipes should take no longer than 15 minutes to prepare and cook. This is based on making full use of our suggestions for some pre-prepared ingredients. If you prefer to prepare your ingredients from scratch then obviously allow longer prep time.

All meat should be trimmed of visible fat and the skin removed.

NUTRITION

All of the recipes in this collection are balanced low calorie meals which should keep you feeling full. It is important to balance your food between proteins, good carbs, good fats, dairy, fruit and vegetables.

Protein. Keeps you feeling full and is also essential for building body tissue. Good protein sources come from meat, fish and eggs.

Carbohydrates. Not all carbs are good and generally they are high in calories, which makes them difficult to include in a calorie limiting diet. However carbs are a good source of energy for your body as they are converted more easily into glucose (sugar) providing energy. Try to eat 'good carbs' which are high in fibre and nutrients e.g. whole fruits and veg, nuts, seeds, whole grain cereals, beans and legumes.

Good Fats. A small amount of fat is an essential part of a healthy, balanced diet. Fat is a source of essential fatty acids such as omega-3 – "essential" because the body can't make them itself. Fat helps the body absorb vitamins A, D and E. Good fats can be found in olive oil, rapeseed oil, avocados, almond nuts and oily fish such as sardines, salmon and tuna.

Dairy. Dairy products provide you with vitamins and minerals. Cheeses can be very high in calories but other products such as low fat Greek yoghurt, crème fraiche and skimmed milk are all good.

Fruit & Vegetables. Eat your five a day. There is never a better time to fill your 5 a day quota. Not only are fruit and veg very healthy, they also fill up your plate and are ideal snacks when you are feeling hungry.

PORTION SIZES

If your goal is weight loss, the size of the portion that you put on your plate will significantly affect your weight loss efforts. Filling your plate with over-sized portions will obviously increase your calorie intake and hamper your dieting efforts.

It's important with all meals that you use a correct sized portion, which generally is the size of your clenched fist. This applies to any side dishes of vegetables and carbs too.

The portion sizes in our 15 Minute Meal recipes are the correct size for the average adult.

THE YOGA PLAN WORKOUTS

Yoga is an ancient form of exercise that focuses on strength, flexibility and breathing. Originating in India more than 5,000 years ago, yoga is practiced to boost physical & mental wellbeing and has been adopted by cultures around the world. It is a safe and effective way to increase physical activity, especially strength, flexibility and balance.

Yoga is thought to have many healing properties and is beneficial for people with high blood pressure, heart disease, aches and pains, depression and stress. There are a number of different types of yoga which are generally practiced including Hatha, Vinyasa & Iyengar to name just three. The routines which have been developed for this book are not confined to one type of yoga and will give you a basic introduction to this wonderful form of exercise. You will find three yoga workouts in this book. The first 2 routines will take around 15 minutes to complete. The third is a 30 minute relaxation session which can be split into two 15 minute routines.

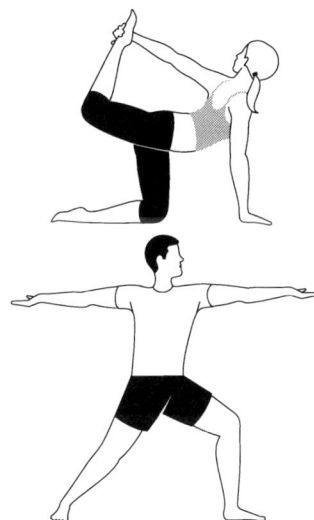

Incorporating a yoga routine into your daily life will benefit you both physically and mentally. All you need to get started is a mat, a block and pillows for support (for the relaxation routine at the end). That said there is no need to run out and buy any equipment at all. You can do any of these routines comfortably on a rug or carpet and the yoga block can be substituted for a small strong shoe sized box.

Yoga will, in time, help you 'still' your mind. When you are doing the routines try to empty your brain of any thoughts. That is not as easy as it sounds, but have patience with yourself. If you try to anchor your thoughts around your breathing you will learn to calm your mind and move towards a stillness which will benefit your well-being.

Enjoy your yoga journey.

YOGA TIPS

- A few things to remember:
- Yoga should never be approached as a competitive sport. It is a personal journey. Always listen to your body and never push yourself too hard. Concentrating on breathing is an extremely important part of yoga practice and you will learnt to use the rhythm of your breathing to help you move through the poses.
- Always move into poses on a breath exhalation and make sure you move slowly and methodically.

ABOUT CookNation

CookNation is the leading publisher of innovative and practical recipe books for the modern, health conscious cook. CookNation titles bring together delicious, easy and practical recipes with their unique approach - easy and delicious, no-nonsense recipes - making cooking for diets and healthy eating fast, simple and fun.

With a range of #1 best-selling titles - from the innovative 'Skinny' calorie-counted series, to the 5:2 Diet Recipes collection - CookNation recipe books prove that 'Diet' can still mean 'Delicious'!

THE *Skinny*
15 MINUTE MEALS
& *YOGA* WORKOUT PLAN

BREAKFAST

MORNING YOGURT

220 calories per serving

Ingredients

- 6 tbsp Greek yogurt
- 1 tsp honey
- 1 tsp green Matcha tea
- 6 walnut halves
- 100g/3½oz strawberries, chopped

Method

1 Combine together the yogurt, honey and matcha tea.

2 Rinse the strawberries, remove the green tops and finely chop, along with the walnuts.

3 Sprinkle both onto the yogurt and serve.

CHEFS NOTE
Try using vanilla yogurt and cut out the honey.

BLUEBERRY PANCAKE

399
calories per serving

Ingredients

- 120ml/½ cup milk
- 1 medium free-range egg
- Pinch of salt
- 50g/2oz buckwheat flour
- 50g/2oz blueberries
- 2 tsp butter
- 1 tbsp Greek yogurt

Method

1 Beat together the milk, egg and salt.

2 Place the buckwheat in another bowl.

3 Gradually add milk mixture to the flour and stir until you get a smooth batter.

4 Add the butter to a hot pan, pour in the mixture and cook for 1-2 minutes on each side, or until golden.

5 Remove from the pan and place to one side while you cook the others.

6 Serve with a dollop of yogurt and the blueberries on top.

CHEFS NOTE
Buckwheat is actually a fruit seed not a cereal grain.

MUSTARD MUSHROOMS ON RYE

265
calories per serving

Ingredients

- 2 tsp olive oil
- ½ garlic cloves, crushed
- 2 shallots, sliced
- 125g/5oz mushrooms, sliced
- 2 tsp Dijon mustard
- 2 tbsp crème fraiche
- 1 piece natural rye bread, lightly toasted
- 1 tbsp freshly chopped flat leaf parsley
- Salt & pepper to taste

Method

1 Gently heat the oil in a pan and sauté the onions and garlic for a few minutes. Add the mushrooms and continue cooking for 8-10 minutes or until the mushrooms are soft and cooked through.

2 Stir through the mustard and crème fraiche, combine well and warm through.

3 Pile the creamy mushrooms and onions onto the rye toast and sprinkle with chopped parsley. Season and serve.

CHEFS NOTE
Add a little paprika to the sauce if you wish.

SERVES 1

WILTED SPINACH & BREAKFAST EGGS

277 calories per serving

Ingredients

- **1 red pepper, deseeded & sliced**
- **½ tsp paprika**
- **2 large free-range eggs**
- **2 tsp olive oil**
- **75g/3oz spinach leaves**
- **Salt & pepper to taste**

Method

1 Break the eggs into a bowl. Add the paprika, a little seasoning and lightly beat with a fork.

2 Gently heat the oil in a frying pan and add the peppers. Sauté for a few minutes until they begin to soften.

3 Add the spinach and allow to wilt for a minute or two. Pour in the beaten eggs and move around the pan until the eggs begin to scramble. As soon as they start to set remove from the heat and serve with lots of black pepper.

CHEFS NOTE
You can turn this into a spicy alternative by adding a little ground chilli, cumin and coriander.

BERRY & CHIA SEED SMOOTHIE

160 calories per serving

Ingredients

- 50g/2oz strawberries
- A small handful of spinach
- 50g/2oz blueberries
- 250ml/1 cup almond milk
- 1 tsp chia seeds
- 1 tbsp Greek yogurt

Method

1 Remove the strawberry tops and any thick stalks from the spinach.

2 Blend all the ingredients together and serve immediately.

CHEFS NOTE
You could also add a handful of ice to this smoothie if you wish.

MANGO & AVOCADO BREAKFAST SALAD

295 calories per serving

Ingredients

- ½ ripe avocado, peeled, stoned & cubed
- ½ ripe mango, peeled, stoned & cubed
- 3 plum tomatoes, diced
- ½ tsp paprika
- ½ red onion, finely chopped
- ½ red chilli, deseeded & finely chopped
- 2 tsp lime juice
- 1 tsp freshly chopped coriander
- 50g/2oz watercress or rocket leaves
- Salt & pepper to taste

Method

1 Combine the cubed avocado, mango, tomatoes, paprika, onions, chilli, lime & coriander together. Allow to sit for a few minutes to let the flavour infuse.

2 Pile onto a bed of watercress or rocket leaves, season & serve.

CHEFS NOTE

Stone the avocados by cutting in half (you'll need to work around the centre stone). When halved, dig the point of the knife into the stone to lever it out, then use a large spoon to scoop each half of the avocado out in one piece.

SCRAMBLED VEGETABLE OMELETTE

345 calories per serving

Ingredients

- 100g/3½oz baby new potatoes, halved
- 75g/3oz tenderstem broccoli, roughly chopped
- 1 tsp olive oil
- ½ onion, sliced
- ½ tsp turmeric & paprika
- Pinch of chilli powder
- 2 large free-range eggs
- Salt & pepper to taste

Method

1 Place the potatoes and chopped broccoli in salted boiling water. Boil for 4-6 minutes or until the potatoes are tender. Drain and put to one side.

2 Meanwhile gently heat the olive oil in a frying pan and sauté the onions for a few minutes until softened. Add the potatoes, broccoli & dried spices to the pan and stir. Cook for a minute or two longer before adding the eggs to the pan.

3 Increase the heat and cook until the eggs are scrambled. Check the seasoning & serve immediately.

CHEFS NOTE
You could also try this recipe substituting the turmeric for ground coriander and garnishing with fresh chopped coriander leaves.

PARMESAN & ROASTED PEPPER FRITTATA

390 calories per serving

Ingredients

- 1 tsp olive oil
- ½ onion, chopped
- 75g/3oz courgettes, sliced
- 75g/3oz roasted peppers, drained & chopped
- 3 free-range eggs
- 1 tsp grated Parmesan cheese
- 2 tsp freshly chopped flat leaf parsley
- Salt & pepper to taste

Method

1 Heat the oil in a frying pan and gently sauté the onions and courgettes for a few minutes until softened. Add the peppers and continue to cook for 2-3 minutes longer.

2 Break the eggs into a bowl and combine with Parmesan cheese. Tip the softened onions and courgettes into the bowl. Mix well and return the eggs & vegetables to the pan, tilting to ensure the mixture covers the base evenly.

3 Cover the pan, reduce the heat and leave to cook for a few minutes. Flip the frittata over and cook the other side until the eggs set and the vegetables are tender.

4 Cut into wedges and serve with chopped parsley sprinkled over the top.

CHEFS NOTE

To keep things really simple use jars of pre-cooked roasted peppers for this recipe.

VICTORIAN BREAKFAST

385 calories per serving

Ingredients

- 2 fresh lambs' kidneys
- 1 tsp olive oil
- 1 garlic clove, crushed
- 75g/3oz button mushrooms, halved
- ½ onion, sliced
- 2 tsp Worcestershire sauce
- ½ tsp cayenne pepper
- 60ml/¼ cup low fat crème fraiche
- 50g/2oz spinach leaves
- 1 English breakfast muffin, lightly toasted
- Salt & pepper to taste

Method

1 Prepare the lambs' kidneys by cutting in half and trimming out any tough core.

2 Gently sauté the garlic, mushrooms & onions for a few minutes until softened.

3 Add the kidneys, Worcestershire sauce and cayenne pepper to the pan. Combine well and cook the kidneys for approx. 4-5 minutes each side.

4 When the kidneys are cooked through, stir in the crème fraiche and spinach and warm through.

5 Season and serve on the toasted English muffin.

CHEFS NOTE

Lambs' kidneys are a traditional breakfast often served during the Victorian era - the spinach is a contemporary addition!

EGGS & MUSHROOMS

240
calories per
serving

Ingredients

- 1 tbsp low fat soft cheese
- 2 tsp freshly chopped chives
- 1 garlic clove, crushed
- 2 large flat mushrooms

- 1 large free-range eggs
- 1 handful rocket leaves
- Salt & pepper to taste

Method

1 Preheat the oven grill.

2 Mix the soft cheese, chives & garlic together and spread evenly on the underside of each mushroom. Season well and place, underside up, under the grill for 5-7 minutes or until the mushrooms are cooked through.

3 Meanwhile fill a frying pan with boiling water and break the eggs into the gently simmering pan to poach while the mushrooms cook.

4 Put the mushrooms on the plates. Arrange the rocket over the top and add a poached egg.

5 Serve with lots of black pepper.

CHEFS NOTE
You can buy low fat soft cheese with chives already added.

THE *Skinny*
15 MINUTE MEALS
&*YOGA* *WORKOUT* PLAN

LUNCH

FRESH SALAD BROTH

160 calories per serving

Ingredients

- 1 tbsp olive oil
- 1 garlic clove, crushed
- 1 onion, sliced
- 1 carrot, diced
- 150g/5oz potatoes, peeled & diced
- 2 tsp dried mixed herbs
- 1lt/4 cups chicken or vegetable stock
- 150g/5oz watercress, roughly chopped
- Salt & pepper to taste

Method

1 Heat the olive oil in a pan and gently sauté the garlic, sliced onions, carrots, potatoes & dried herbs for a few minutes until softened. Add the stock, bring to the boil, cover and leave to simmer for 10 minutes or until everything is tender.

2 Blend to your preferred consistency and add the watercress.

3 Stir through, season and serve immediately.

CHEFS NOTE

Any mix of dried herbs will work well with this light summery soup. This soup serves 4 and can be stored in the fridge or freezer.

ASPARAGUS & PORTABELLA OPEN SANDWICH

280 calories per serving

Ingredients

- 2 tsp olive oil
- 8 asparagus spears, chopped
- 1 large portabella mushroom, sliced
- ½ onion, sliced
- ½ tsp dried basil
- 1 tsp lemon juice
- Pinch of crushed chilli flakes
- 2 tsp freshly chopped flat leaf parsley
- ½ ciabatta roll
- Salt & pepper to taste

Method

1 Heat the olive oil in a pan and gently sauté the asparagus, mushroom, onions & basil for a few minutes until softened.

2 Meanwhile gently toast the ciabatta half.

3 When the mushrooms and asparagus are tender add the lemon juice and chilli flakes. Stir through, season and serve on top of the toasted ciabatta with the chopped parsley sprinkled on top.

CHEFS NOTE
Add a little water during sautéing if the pan needs loosening up.

PARMESAN CRUSTED SALMON

410 calories per serving

Ingredients

- 150g/5oz baby new potatoes, halved
- 1 boneless, skinless salmon fillet weighing 125g/4oz
- 2 tsp grated Parmesan cheese
- 1 tbsp fresh breadcrumbs
- 1 garlic clove, crushed
- 100g/3 ½oz tenderstem broccoli
- Lemon wedges to serve
- Salt & pepper to taste

Method

1 Cook the new potatoes in a pan of salted boiling water until tender.

2 Meanwhile season the salmon fillet. Mix the Parmesan cheese, breadcrumbs & garlic together and coat the top of the salmon fillet with the breadcrumb mixture.

3 Place the salmon under a preheated grill and cook for 10 minutes or until the salmon fillets are cooked through.

4 Whilst the salmon and potatoes are cooking plunge the broccoli into salted boiling water and cook for a 2-3 minutes or until tender.

5 Drain the potatoes and broccoli and serve with the salmon fillets and lemon wedges.

CHEFS NOTE

To make fresh breadcrumbs place a slice of bread in the food processor and pulse for a few seconds.

SERVES 4

MUSHROOM & CARAMELISED ONION SOUP

190 calories per serving

Ingredients

- 1 tsp olive oil
- 2 garlic cloves, crushed
- 2 onions, chopped
- 2 tbsp balsamic vinegar
- 200g/7oz potatoes, peeled & diced
- 500g/1lb 2oz mushrooms, sliced
- 1ltml/4 cups vegetable stock/broth
- Salt & pepper to taste

Method

1 Heat the oil in a saucepan and add the garlic, onions & balsamic vinegar. Sauté on a high heat until the onions are cooked crispy brown and the balsamic vinegar reduces down. Put to one side when caramelised.

2 Meanwhile add the potatoes, mushrooms & stock to a saucepan. Bring to the boil and simmer for 8-10 minutes or until the potatoes are soft.

3 Blend to a smooth consistency and divide into bowls.

4 Split the onions equally and place in the centre of each bowl of soup. Season and serve.

CHEFS NOTE
This soup serves 4 and can be stored in the fridge or freezer. Add some chopped chives if you like and serve with crusty bread!

27

CHICKEN NOODLE RAMEN

380 calories per serving

Ingredients

- 1 leek, sliced
- 1 celery stalk, chopped
- 1 carrot, chopped
- ½ tsp dried thyme
- 250ml/1 cup chicken stock
- 2 spring onions, sliced thinly lengthways
- 125g/4oz cooked chicken breast, shredded
- 75g/3oz tinned sweetcorn, drained
- 100g/3½oz straight-to-wok wholewheat ramen noodles
- Salt & pepper to taste

Method

1 Place the leeks, celery and carrots in a saucepan along with the thyme and stock. Bring to the boil and simmer for 7-10 minutes or until all the vegetables are soft.

2 Blend to a smooth consistency and return to the pan. Add the shredded chicken, sweetcorn & noodles and cook for a further 4-6 minutes or until the ramen is piping hot.

3 Check the seasoning and serve with the sliced spring onions on top.

CHEFS NOTE
Dried noodles are fine to use too. Just use half the quantity and cook for a little longer in the stock.

WARM CUCUMBER TUNA SALAD

220
calories per serving

Ingredients

- ¼ cucumber, finely sliced into matchsticks
- ½-1 tsp caster sugar
- 1-2 tbsp rice wine vinegar
- Pinch of dried chilli flakes
- 100g/3½oz tinned borlotti beans, drained & rinsed
- 50g/2oz cherry tomatoes, halved
- ½ red onion, finely chopped
- 100g/3½oz tinned tuna, drained
- 75g/3oz rocket
- Salt & pepper to taste

Method

1 Place the cucumber in a frying pan and gently warm over a low heat.

2 Add the caster sugar, rice wine vinegar & chilli flakes. Simmer for a few minutes and set aside to cool.

3 Meanwhile mix together the red onion, beans, tomatoes & tuna in a large bowl. Add the cooled cucumber, toss with the rocket and serve.

CHEFS NOTE
This is a simple Asian salad. You may need to balance the sugar and vinegar a little.

LEMON & BASIL ZUCCHINI GNOCCHI

405 calories per serving

Ingredients

- 2 tsp olive oil
- 1 garlic clove, crushed
- 125g/5oz baby courgettes, thinly sliced lengthways
- 1 tbsp lemon juice
- 1 tbsp freshly chopped basil
- 150g/5oz gnocchi
- Salt & pepper to taste

Method

1 Gently heat the olive oil in a frying pan and sauté the garlic, courgettes, lemon juice & basil.

2 Meanwhile place the gnocchi in a pan of salted boiling water. Cook for 2-3 minutes or until the gnocchi begins to float to the top. As soon as the gnocchi is cooked, drain and place in the frying pan with the courgettes on a high heat.

3 Move the gnocchi around for a minute or two to coat each dumpling in oil. Season and serve.

CHEFS NOTE
Spinach also makes a nice addition to this veggie dish.

PARSLEY & PARMESAN SPIRALS

SERVES 1

Ingredients

- 1 large courgette/zucchini
- 1 tbsp extra virgin olive oil
- 1 garlic clove, crushed
- 2 shallots, sliced
- 1 tsp lemon juice
- 2 tbsp freshly chopped flat leaf parsley
- 1 tbsp grated Parmesan cheese
- Salt & pepper to taste

Method

1 First spiralize the courgette into thick spirals.

2 Heat the olive oil in a high-sided frying pan and gently sauté the garlic and shallots for a few minutes. Add the courgette spirals and increase the heat. Stir fry for 2-3 minutes.

3 Remove from the heat. Add the lemon juice, parsley and Parmesan. Toss well, season & serve.

CHEFS NOTE

You will need a Spiralizer for this dish if you don't have one, pre-prepared shredded vegetables are now available in most supermarkets.

TENDER BROCCOLI WITH ANCHOVY DRESSING

255 calories per serving

Ingredients

- 4 tinned anchovy fillets
- 200g/7oz tenderstem broccoli
- 1 tbsp olive oil
- 1 garlic clove, crushed
- ½ onion, finely sliced
- ½ red chilli, deseeded & finely chopped
- Salt & pepper to taste

Method

1 Drain the anchovy fillets and put to one side.

2 Plunge the broccoli into a pan of salted boiling water and cook for 2 minutes. Drain and put to one side.

3 Heat the olive oil in a frying pan and gently sauté the garlic, onion, chilli, and anchovy fillets and cook for a few minutes until anchovies begin to break up.

4 Add the broccoli to the pan and increase the heat. Toss until well combined.

5 Check the seasoning and serve.

CHEFS NOTE
Tenderstem broccoli is great for making quick lunches and suppers. Use crushed chillies if you don't have fresh chillies to hand.

CHICKPEA PRAWN BOWL

SERVES 1

420 calories per serving

Ingredients

- 1 tbsp olive oil
- ½ onion, sliced
- 1 garlic cloves, crushed
- ½ red chilli, deseeded & finely chopped
- 100g/3½oz ripe plum tomatoes, roughly chopped
- 200g/7oz tinned chickpeas, drained
- 150g/5oz peeled raw king prawns
- 2 tsp lemon juice
- 1 tbsp freshly chopped parsley
- Lemon wedges to serve
- Salt & pepper to taste

Method

1 Heat the olive in a pan and gently sauté the onion, garlic & chilli for a few minutes until softened.

2 Add the roughly chopped tomatoes, chickpeas & prawns and leave to gently simmer for 10 minutes stirring occasionally. Add the lemon juice and combine well.

3 Cover and simmer for a further couple of minutes or until the prawns are pink and cooked through. Sprinkle with chopped basil and serve with lemon wedges.

CHEFS NOTE
Try serving with leafy greens or wild rice.

CITRUS HERB BULGUR SALAD

260 calories per serving

Ingredients

- 50g/2oz bulgur wheat
- 1 tbsp pine nuts
- ½ onion, chopped
- ½ garlic clove, crushed
- 1 tbsp lime juice
- 1 tbsp olive oil
- 1 bunch spring onions/scallions, sliced lengthways
- Lime wedges to serve
- 2 tbsp freshly chopped mixed herbs
- 1 romaine lettuce, shredded
- Salt & pepper to taste

Method

1 Cook the bulgur wheat in salted boiling water for 10 minutes or until tender.

2 Place the pine nuts in a dry frying pan and lightly toast for a minute or two.

3 Put to one side and use the same pan to gently sauté the chopped onions & garlic for a few minutes.

4 Add the lime juice, fluff the bulgar with a fork and pile into the onion pan along with the toasted pine nuts. Mix well, and serve over the shredded lettuce with fresh lime wedges on the side and the herbs & spring onions sprinkled over the top.

CHEFS NOTE
This simple dish is lovely served alone but is a great side to grilled tuna too.

FRESH SARDINES

330
calories per serving

Ingredients

- 2 fresh sardines each weighing 125g/4oz
- 1 garlic clove, crushed
- 2 tsp extra virgin olive oil
- 1 tsp lemon juice
- Large pinch of paprika
- 1 tbsp freshly chopped oregano
- Lemon wedges to serve
- Salt & pepper to taste

Method

1 Preheat the grill to a medium/high heat.

2 Ask your fishmonger to prepare the sardines by gutting, cleaning & boning them for you. Mix together the garlic, olive oil, lemon juice & paprika and brush onto either side of each fish.

3 Place the sardines under the grill and cook for 4-5 minutes each side or until the sardines are cooked through. Remove from the grill, season and serve with lemon wedges and oregano sprinkled over the top.

CHEFS NOTE
These lightly dressed sardines are also easy to cook on the barbeque.

PAN FRIED LEMON & PAPRIKA HADDOCK

290
calories per serving

Ingredients

- **1 boneless, skinless haddock fillet weighing 150g/5oz**
- **½ onion, sliced**
- **125g/4oz mushrooms**
- **¼ tsp each paprika & mixed spice**
- **1 tsp lemon juice**
- **2 tsp olive oil**
- **150g/5oz rocket**
- **Salt & pepper to taste**

Method

1 Season the haddock fillet.

2 Gently sauté the garlic in the olive oil for a few minutes. Add the onions, mushrooms, paprika, mixed spice & lemon juice and cook for 5 minutes or until the onions are softened.

3 Move the vegetables to one side of the pan to make room for the haddock fillets. Cook for 3-5 minutes each side depending on the thickness of the fillet, or until cooked through.

4 Serve the cooked haddock fillet on a bed of rocket with the onions & mushrooms arranged over the top of the fish.

CHEFS NOTE

Serve with lemon wedges and chopped parsley if you wish.

CREAMY LEEK & POTATO SOUP

210
calories per serving

Ingredients

- 500g/1lb 2oz potatoes
- 500g/1lb 2oz leeks
- 1lt/4 cups vegetable stock/broth
- 60ml/¼ cup low fat single cream
- Salt & pepper to taste

Method

1 Peel and chop the potatoes & leeks.

2 Place the potatoes and leeks in a saucepan with the hot stock. Bring to the boil and leave to simmer for 10-12 minutes or until the potatoes and tender.

3 Blend the soup to a smooth consistency, stir through the cream, check the seasoning and serve.

CHEFS NOTE
This soup serves 4 and can be stored in the fridge or freezer.

HORSERADISH MACKEREL & SPINACH

350 calories per serving

Ingredients

- 1 fresh, boned headless mackerel weighing 150g/5oz
- 1 tsp curry powder
- 1 tsp olive oil
- 2 tsp horseradish sauce
- 1 tsp lemon juice
- 1 tsp chopped capers
- 125g/5oz spinach
- Salt & pepper to taste

Method

1 Butterfly the mackerel to open into one large flat fillet. Season the fish and rub with curry powder.

2 Heat the olive oil in a pan and fry the mackerel for 3 minutes each side.

3 Meanwhile combine together the horseradish sauce, lemon juice & capers to make a dressing.

4 When the fish is cooked, wrap in foil and put to one side to keep warm. Add the spinach to the empty pan and cook for a few minutes. Stir the dressing through the wilted spinach and serve with the cooked mackerel fillets.

CHEFS NOTE

Use shop-bought horseradish or make your own my combining freshly grated horseradish, crème fraiche, lemon juice & Dijon mustard.

ALMOND & ONION SPROUT SALAD

270 calories per serving

Ingredients

- 150g/5oz prepared Brussels sprouts
- 1 tbsp olive oil
- 1 onions, sliced
- 50g/2oz blanched almonds
- Salt & pepper to taste

Method

1 Slice the sprouts really thinly so they fall into shreds.

2 Heat the olive oil in a frying pan and gently sauté the onions for 8-10 minutes or until they are soft and golden.

3 Meanwhile plunge the shredded sprouts into salted boiling water for 2 minutes. Drain and rinse through with cold water. Add to the onion pan along with the almonds and toss until piping hot and cooked through.

4 Season with plenty of salt & freshly ground pepper to serve.

CHEFS NOTE
To blanch almonds: place the almonds in a bowl of boiling water for one minute. Drain & rinse under cold water. Pat dry and slip off their skins.

CHILLI PRAWNS & MANGO

410 calories per serving

Ingredients

- 125g/4oz wholemeal microwavable rice
- ½ red pepper, deseeded & sliced
- ½ onion, sliced
- 1 garlic clove, crushed
- 1 tsp freshly grated ginger
- ½ tsp brown sugar
- 1 tsp olive oil

- 1 tsp soy sauce
- 150g/5oz shelled raw king prawns
- Pinch of dried chilli flakes
- ½ mango, stoned & finely chopped
- 1 tbsp freshly chopped coriander
- 2 tsp lime juice
- Salt & pepper to taste

Method

1 Gently sauté the sliced peppers, onions, garlic, ginger & sugar in the olive oil for a few minutes until softened.

2 Add the prawns & chilli flakes and cook for 5-8 minutes or until the prawns are pink and cooked through.

3 Add the rice to the pan, combine well and cook together for a minute or two longer.

4 Combine together the mango, coriander and lime juice to make a mango salsa.

5 Place prawns and rice into a bowl and serve with the mango salsa piled on top.

CHEFS NOTE
Microwavable rice is also suitable for stir frying as it's already cooked and just needs warming through.

RYE & PARMESAN CRUSTED SALMON

440
calories per serving

Ingredients

- 50g/2oz bulgur wheat
- 1 boneless, skinless salmon fillet weighing 150g/5oz
- 2 tsp grated Parmesan cheese
- 1 tbsp fresh rye breadcrumbs
- ½ garlic clove, crushed
- 200g/7oz tenderstem broccoli
- Lemon wedges to serve
- Salt & pepper to taste

Method

1 Cook the bulgur wheat in salted boiling water for 15 minutes or until tender.

2 Meanwhile season the salmon fillet. Mix the Parmesan cheese, breadcrumbs & garlic together and coat the top of the salmon fillet with the breadcrumb mixture.

3 Place the salmon under a preheated grill and cook for 10-13 minutes or until the salmon fillets are cooked through.

4 Whilst the salmon is cooking plunge the broccoli into salted boiling water and cook for a 2-3 minutes or until tender.

5 Drain any excess liquid from the bulgur wheat and fluff with a fork. Drain the broccoli and serve with the salmon fillet, bulgur wheat and lemon wedges.

CHEFS NOTE

To make fresh breadcrumbs place a slice of rye bread in the food processor and pulse for a few seconds.

SIMPLE BROCCOLI & CAULIFLOWER SOUP

168 calories per serving

Ingredients

- 75g/3oz cauliflower florets, chopped
- 75g/3oz broccoli florets, chopped
- 100g/3½oz tinned cooked lentils
- 1 shallot, chopped

- 1 tbsp chopped flat leaf parsley
- 250ml/1 cups vegetable stock/broth
- 120ml/½ cup milk
- Salt & pepper to taste

Method

1 Add all the ingredients, except the milk, to the saucepan.

2 Bring to the boil and leave to gently simmer for 8-10 minutes or until the vegetables are tender.

3 Blend to a smooth consistency, add the milk, and heat through for a minute or two. Check the seasoning and serve with freshly chopped parsley sprinkled over the top.

CHEFS NOTE
Cooked lentils are widely available and are a great time saver.

SPICED MACKEREL FILLET

460 calories per serving

Ingredients

- 1 fresh, boned headless mackerel weighing 150g/5oz
- 1 tsp curry powder
- 1 tsp olive oil
- 1 tbsp horseradish sauce
- 1 tsp lemon juice
- 1 tsp chopped capers
- 100g/3½oz spinach
- Salt & pepper to taste

Method

1 Butterfly the mackerel to open into one large flat fillet. Season and rub with the curry powder.

2 Heat the olive oil in a pan and fry the mackerel for 3 minutes each side.

3 Meanwhile combine together the horseradish sauce, lemon juice & capers to make a dressing.

4 When the fish is cooked, wrap in foil and put to one side to keep warm. Add the spinach to the empty pan and cook for a few minutes. Stir the dressing through the wilted spinach and serve with the cooked mackerel fillet.

CHEFS NOTE

Some shop-bought horseradish can be high in salt so make sure you check the ingredients.

COD & CHUNKY SALSA

430 calories per serving

Ingredients

- 1 tsp lime juice
- 1 tsp white wine vinegar
- 6 cherry tomatoes, diced
- 1 spring onions, finely chopped
- ½ avocado, peeled & stoned
- 1 garlic clove, crushed

- 2 tsp olive oil
- 75g/3oz asparagus spears
- 1 boneless, skinless cod fillet weighing 150g/5oz
- 50g/2oz watercress
- Salt & pepper to taste

Method

1 Combine together the lime juice, vinegar, cherry tomatoes, spring onions and avocado to create a chunky salsa.

2 Mix together the garlic & olive oil and brush onto the cod fillet & asparagus spears.

3 Place the fish and asparagus under a preheated grill and cook for 6-9 minutes or until the cod is cooked through and the asparagus spears are tender

4 Season and serve the cooked cod with the salsa over the top and the watercress on the side of the plate.

CHEFS NOTE

Chopped coriander sprinkled over the salsa makes a good addition.

SUNDRIED TOMATO & CHICKEN SALAD

440 calories per serving

Ingredients

- 150g/5oz cooked skinless chicken breast
- 75g/3oz cherry tomatoes
- 3 sundried tomatoes, finely chopped
- 25g/1oz Dolcelatte cheese
- 2 tsp extra virgin olive oil

- 2 tsp cider vinegar
- 1 tbsp crème fraiche
- ½ tsp paprika
- 75g/3oz watercress
- Salt & pepper to taste

Method

1 Slice the cooked chicken into strips and put to one side to cool.

2 Halve the cherry tomatoes and crumble the Dolcelatte cheese.

3 Combine together the olive oil, vinegar, crème fraiche & paprika to make a dressing.

4 Toss the dressing, tomatoes, sundried tomatoes & cheese together in a large bowl and serve on a bed of watercress with the chicken slices on top.

CHEFS NOTE
Feta cheese also works well in this recipe.

OREGANO & CHILLI SPAGHETTI

350 calories per serving

Ingredients

- 75g/3oz wholewheat spaghetti
- 1 tsp dried oregano
- Pinch of crushed chilli flakes
- 1 tsp pitted black olives, chopped
- ½ onion, sliced
- 1 tbsp sundried tomato puree
- 2 tsp olive oil
- Handful of rocket
- Salt & pepper to taste

Method

1 Cook the spaghetti in a pan of salted boiling water until tender.

2 Meanwhile gently sauté the oregano, chilli, olives, onions & sundried tomato puree for a few minutes or until the onions are softened. Drain the cooked pasta and add to the pan.

3 Toss well with the rocket, season & serve.

CHEFS NOTE

If you don't have sundried tomato puree, you could use chopped sundried tomatoes and regular puree.

SICILIAN CAPONATA

345 calories per serving

Ingredients

- 1 tsp olive oil
- 1 aubergine, cubed
- 1 courgettes, sliced in half lengthways
- 1 tsp dried oregano
- ½ onion, sliced
- 1 celery stalk, chopped
- 1 garlic clove, crushed
- 1 tbsp balsamic vinegar
- 1 tsp capers, chopped
- 75g/3oz ripe plum tomatoes, roughly chopped
- 1 tsp pitted black olives, sliced
- 1 tsp sultanas, roughly chopped
- 125g/4oz wholemeal microwavable rice
- Salt & pepper to taste

Method

1 Gently sauté the aubergines, courgettes, oregano, onions, celery and garlic in the olive oil for a few minutes until softened.

2 Add the balsamic vinegar, capers, tomatoes, olives & sultanas and continue to cook for 10 minutes or until everything is cooked through and tender.

3 Add the rice to the pan. Combine well, season & serve.

CHEFS NOTE
Caponata is a southern Italian dish which can also be served cold.

FETA, APPLE & DATE SALAD

Ingredients

- 1 raw beetroot bulb, peeled
- 125g/4oz apple peeled & cored
- 50g/2oz medjool dates, stoned
- 1 tbsp freshly chopped oregano
- 1 tbsp balsamic vinegar
- 1 tbsp extra virgin olive oil
- 50g/2oz feta cheese
- 75g/4oz watercress
- Salt & pepper to taste

Method

1 Grate, or finely chop, the beetroot bulbs – ideally in a food processor.

2 Cut the apple into fine slices, chop the dates and gently combine both with the grated beetroot.

3 Add the oregano, balsamic vinegar & oil to the salad and mix well.

4 Check the seasoning and arrange on a bed of watercress with the feta cheese crumbled over the top.

CHEFS NOTE
Use more or less balsamic vinegar to suit your own taste.

THE *Skinny*
15 MINUTE MEALS
& *YOGA* WORKOUT PLAN

DINNER

CAULIFLOWER & CHIVE RISOTTO

470
calories per serving

Ingredients

- 1 tbsp olive oil
- 1 garlic clove, crushed
- ½ onion, sliced
- 1 celery stalk, finely chopped
- 100g/3½oz quick cook Arborio risotto
- 250ml/1 cup vegetable stock/broth
- ½ head cauliflower
- ½ tsp crushed dried chillies
- 1 tbsp freshly chopped chives
- Salt & pepper to taste

Method

1 Heat the olive oil and gently sauté the onion, celery and garlic for a couple of minutes until softened.

2 Add the risotto rice to the pan and stir well to coat each grain in olive oil. Add a ladle of stock and simmer until the stock is absorbed. Continue cooking the risotto adding a ladle of stock each time and allowing the rice to absorb the stock until adding the next ladle. Continue cooking for about 10 mins or until the rice is tender. Add more water or stock if needed.

3 Meanwhile quarter the cauliflower and place into a food processor. Pulse for a few seconds to make into rice size grains. Add to the risotto along with the crushed chillies. Combine well and continue cooking until the risotto rice and cauliflower 'rice' are both tender. Add the chopped chives, stir well, season and serve.

CHEFS NOTE
The cauliflower will add to the creaminess of this lovely simple dish.

FISH & COUSCOUS

490 calories per serving

Ingredients

- 1 tsp olive oil
- ½ onion, sliced
- 1 garlic clove, crushed
- ½ tsp crushed chilli flakes
- 120ml/½ cup tomato passata/sieved tomatoes
- 200g/7oz skinless, boneless white fish fillet
- 1 tbsp freshly chopped flat leaf parsley
- 370ml/1½ cups fish stock/broth
- 200g/7oz couscous
- Salt & pepper to taste

Method

1 Gently sauté the onion, garlic & chilli in the olive oil for a few minutes until softened. Add the passata, fish & parsley and leave to gently simmer for 8 minutes stirring occasionally.

2 Whilst the fish is cooking, place the couscous in a pan with the hot stock. Bring the pan to the boil, remove from the heat, cover and leave to stand for 3-4 minutes or until all the stock is absorbed and the couscous is tender.

3 Fluff the couscous with a fork and serve into a bowl. Place the fish and sauce piled on the top.

CHEFS NOTE
This poached fish dish is super-simple and quick to make. Be sure to season really well.

SIMPLE SICILIAN GNOCCHI

490
calories per serving

Ingredients

- 250g/9oz gnocchi
- 1 tbsp extra virgin olive oil
- 2 garlic cloves, crushed
- 2 tsp lemon juice
- 1 tbsp freshly chopped flat leaf parsley
- 1 tsp freshly grated Parmesan cheese
- Salt & pepper to taste

Method

1 Place the gnocchi in a pan of salted boiling water. Cook for 2-3 minutes or until the gnocchi begins to float to the top.

2 Meanwhile gently sauté the garlic in the olive oil whilst the gnocchi cooks.

3 Drain the gnocchi and add to the frying pan. Toss well, sprinkle with freshly chopped parsley, season & serve with the grated Parmesan.

CHEFS NOTE
This dish is also good with some fresh peas tossed through at the end of cooking.

CHICKEN & SPINACH PENNE

495 calories per serving

Ingredients

- 100g/3½oz skinless chicken breast, sliced
- 75g/3oz wholewheat penne pasta
- 1 tbsp olive oil
- 1 garlic clove, crushed
- 1 tsp freshly chopped thyme
- 100g/3½oz baby spinach leaves
- 60ml/¼ cup chicken stock
- 1 tsp grated Parmesan
- Salt & pepper to taste

Method

1 Heat the olive oil in a frying pan and begin cooking the sliced chicken for 3-4 minutes. Meanwhile cook the penne in a pan of salted boiling water until tender.

2 Add the garlic, thyme, spinach & stock and cook until everything is tender and piping hot. Drain the cooked penne and add to the frying pan.

3 Toss well and serve with the grated Parmesan sprinkled on top.

CHEFS NOTE
Try using rosemary or oregano if you like. Dried herbs are fine to use if you don't have fresh herbs to hand.

ITALIAN CHICKEN & BEANS

490 calories per serving

Ingredients

- 2 tsp olive oil
- 1 onion, sliced
- ½ fennel bulb, finely sliced
- 1 garlic clove, crushed
- 250g/9oz tinned flageolet beans, drained
- 150g/5oz skinless chicken breast, thickly sliced
- 120ml/½ cup chicken stock/broth
- 1 tbsp freshly chopped basil
- Salt & pepper to taste

Method

1 Gently sauté the onion, fennel and garlic in the olive oil for a few minutes until softened.

2 Add the beans, chicken & stock and leave to gently simmer for 10 minutes or until the chicken is cooked through and the stock has reduced.

3 Sprinkle with chopped basil, season and serve.

CHEFS NOTE
Borlotti or cannellini beans will work just as well for this dish.

PORCINI & THYME LINGUINE

390 calories per serving

Ingredients

- 25g/1oz dried porcini mushrooms
- 75g/3oz wholemeal linguine
- 1 tsp olive oil
- 1 garlic clove, crushed
- ½ onion, sliced
- 1 tsp dried thyme
- 1 tbsp low fat mascarpone cheese
- 1 tsp tomato puree
- Salt & pepper to taste

Method

1 Place the porcini mushrooms in a little boiling water and leave to rehydrate for a few minutes. Thinly slice when softened.

2 Cook the spaghetti in a pan of salted boiling water until tender.

3 Meanwhile heat the olive oil in a high-sided frying pan and gently sauté the garlic, onions & dried thyme whilst the pasta cooks.

4 When the onions are soft add the mascarpone cheese, and tomato puree and stir well. Drain the cooked pasta and add to the frying pan.

5 Toss well. Season & serve.

CHEFS NOTE
Dried porcini mushrooms are readily available in any supermarket.

PRAWN & CHORIZO ANGEL HAIR PASTA

395 calories per serving

Ingredients

- 75g/3oz wholemeal angel hair pasta
- 1 tbsp olive oil
- 1 garlic clove, crushed
- 25g/1oz chorizo, finely chopped or sliced
- ½ tsp paprika

- ½ onion, sliced
- 150g/5oz shelled raw king prawns, chopped
- 2 tsp lemon juice
- 1 tsp freshly chopped flat leaf parsley
- Salt & pepper to taste

Method

1 Cook the spaghetti in a pan of salted boiling water until tender.

2 Meanwhile heat the olive oil in a high-sided frying pan and gently sauté the garlic, chorizo, paprika and onions for 5 minutes whilst the pasta cooks.

3 Add the chopped prawns and lemon juice and cook until the prawns are pink and cooked through. Drain the cooked pasta, add to the frying pan and combine really well.

4 Sprinkle with chopped parsley and serve.

CHEFS NOTE
Chorizo and shellfish are a classic combination. Serve with lots of freshly ground black pepper.

COD, ASPARAGUS & AVOCADO

480 calories per serving

Ingredients

- 1 garlic clove, crushed
- 2 tsp olive oil
- 100g/3½oz asparagus spears
- 1 boneless, skinless cod fillet weighing 150g/5oz
- 150g/5oz ripe plum tomatoes, finely chopped
- Bunch spring onions, finely chopped
- ½ avocado peeled, stoned & cubed
- 2 tsp freshly chopped oregano
- 75g/3oz watercress
- 1 tsp lime juice
- Salt & pepper to taste

Method

1 Mix together the garlic & olive oil and brush onto the cod fillet & asparagus spears.

2 Place the fish and asparagus under a preheated grill and cook for 5-7 minutes or until the cod is cooked through and the asparagus spears are tender

3 Meanwhile combine the chopped tomatoes, spring onions, avocado, lime, chopped oregano & watercress together.

4 Season and serve the cooked cod with the watercress tomato salad.

CHEFS NOTE
Any firm white fish will work just as well for this dish.

STEAK & STILTON SAUCE

450
calories per serving

Ingredients

- 175g/6oz sweet potatoes
- 1 sirloin steak weighing 125g/4oz
- 1 tsp olive oil
- 75g/3oz fresh peas

- 25g/1oz stilton cheese
- 1 tbsp crème fraiche
- 60ml/¼ cup chicken stock
- Salt & pepper to taste

Method

1 Peel the sweet potatoes, cut into 1cm slices and cook in the saucepan for 10-12 minutes or until they are tender.

2 Meanwhile trim any fat off the steak. Season and brush with the olive oil while you put a frying pan on a high heat.

3 Place the steak in the smoking hot dry pan and cook for 1-2 minutes each side, or to your liking.

4 When the steak is cooked put to one side to rest for 3 minutes.

5 Whilst the steak is resting, quickly cook the peas in salted boiling water for a minute or two. In a separate pan gently heat and stir the stilton, crème fraiche and stock to make a sauce.

6 Serve the steak, sweet potatoes & fresh peas with the stilton sauce drizzled over the top.

CHEFS NOTE
Adjust the steak cooking time depending on your preference and the thickness of the cut.

EGG MOLEE

450 calories per serving

Ingredients

- 125g/4oz wholemeal microwavable rice
- 1 garlic clove, crushed
- ½ onion, chopped
- 75g/3oz peas
- 1 tsp olive oil
- 2 tsp tomato puree
- ½ tsp each turmeric, garam masala & ground ginger
- 60ml/¼ cup low fat coconut milk
- 2 large free-range hard boiled eggs
- Salt & pepper to taste

Method

1 Gently sauté the garlic, onions & peas in the olive oil for a few minutes until softened.

2 Stir through the tomato puree, dried spices & coconut milk until combined. Cut the eggs in half and place yolk side up, in the coconut milk. Gently cook until warmed through.

3 When everything is piping hot, cook the rice and spoon the curry on top.

4 Season and serve.

CHEFS NOTE

To hard boil the eggs place in cold water. Bring to the boil and cook for four minutes. Remove from the heat, allow to cool and peel.

TUNA STEAK & SPICED COURGETTES

320 calories per serving

Ingredients

- 2 courgettes, diced
- ½ red onion, finely chopped
- 2 tsp olive oil
- 1 fresh tuna steak weighing 150g/5oz
- 1 tbsp balsamic vinegar
- 100g/3½oz watercress
- Salt & pepper to taste

Method

1 Gently sauté the courgettes and red onion in 1 tsp of the olive oil for a few minutes until softened.

2 Season the tuna and put a frying pan on a high heat with the rest of the olive oil and balsamic vinegar.

3 Place the tuna in the pan and cook for 2 minutes each side. Remove the tuna from the pan and serve with the watercress and courgette side dish.

CHEFS NOTE
Two minutes of cooking each side should leave the tuna rare in the centre. Reduce or increase cooking time depending on your preference.

LEMON & OLIVE PENNE

430
calories per
serving

Ingredients

- 75g/3oz wholemeal penne
- 1 tsp olive oil
- ½ onion, sliced
- 1 garlic clove, crushed
- 1 tbsp pitted black olives, sliced
- 1 tsp balsamic vinegar
- 1 tbsp lemon juice
- 1 tbsp freshly chopped basil
- 50g/2oz low fat mozzarella cheese, cubed
- Salt & pepper to taste

Method

1 Cook the penne in a pan of salted boiling water until tender.

2 Meanwhile heat the olive oil in a high-sided frying pan and gently sauté the onions & garlic for 3-4 minutes. Add the olives, balsamic vinegar & lemon juice and cook until everything is tender and piping hot.

3 Drain the cooked penne and add to the frying pan along with the cubed mozzarella cheese. Stir through until the cheese melts.

4 Season and serve.

CHEFS NOTE
Make sure you serve this dish when it is still nice and hot so that the mozzarella cheese remains melted.

CREAMY PARMA PASTA

440 calories per serving

Ingredients

- 1 tsp olive oil
- ½ onion, sliced
- 50g/2oz peas
- 2 slices Parma ham, chopped
- 2 tbsp low fat crème fraiche

- 75g/3oz wholewheat fusilli
- 1 tbsp freshly chopped flat leaf parsley
- 1 tsp grated Parmesan cheese
- Salt & pepper to taste

Method

1 Cook the fusilli and peas in a pan of salted boiling water until tender.

2 Meanwhile heat the olive oil in a high-sided frying pan and gently sauté the onions for a few minutes. When the onions are softened remove from the pan, increase the heat and add the chopped Parma ham. Cook until crispy, reduce the heat and return the onions to the pan along with the crème fraiche.

3 Drain the cooked pasta and add to the frying pan along with the Parmesan cheese.

4 Toss well and serve with the chopped parsley on top.

CHEFS NOTE

You could stir the parsley though the sauce rather than using as a garnish if you prefer.

ASIAN CHICKEN SALAD

240 calories per serving

Ingredients

- 1 tsp honey
- 1 tbsp soy sauce
- 1 tsp olive oil
- 1 tsp rice wine vinegar
- ½ garlic clove, crushed
- 1 tsp freshly grated ginger
- 125g/4oz cooked chicken breast, sliced
- ½ red chilli, deseeded & finely chopped
- ½ cucumber, sliced into batons
- 1 carrot, thinly sliced into ribbons
- 2 spring onions, thinly sliced lengthways
- ½ large romaine lettuces shredded
- 1 tbsp freshly chopped coriander
- Salt & pepper to taste

Method

1 Mix together the honey, soy sauce, olive oil, rice wine vinegar, garlic and ginger to make a dressing.

2 Place the chicken, chilli, cucumber, carrots and spring onions into a large bowl and combine well with the dressing.

3 Arrange the shredded lettuce on four plates and pile the dressed chicken and vegetables on top. Sprinkle with chopped coriander & serve.

CHEFS NOTE
Use a vegetable peeler to cut the carrots into very thin ribbons.

BROAD BEAN & OREGANO LENTILS

390 calories per serving

Ingredients

- 200g/7oz cooked tinned lentils
- 200g/7oz shelled fresh broad beans
- 2 tsp olive oil
- 3 anchovy fillets, drained
- ½ garlic clove, crushed
- 2 shallots, sliced
- 100g/3½oz ripe plum tomatoes, roughly chopped
- 1 tbsp freshly chopped oregano
- 50g/2oz rocket
- Salt & pepper to taste

Method

1 Place the broad beans in a pan of boiling water, cook for 2 minutes and drain.

2 Meanwhile heat the olive oil in a high-sided frying pan and gently sauté the anchovy fillets, garlic, onions, chopped tomatoes and oregano. Once cooked, leave to cool.

3 Drain the lentils and toss well with the cooled tomato mix.

4 Pile onto top of a bed or rocket and serve.

CHEFS NOTE
Try garnishing this with some extra fresh tomatoes, raw red onions and chopped basil.

SERVES 1

SPICY MUSSELS

305 calories per serving

Ingredients

- 500g/1lb 2oz mussels
- 1 tbsp olive oil
- ½ garlic clove, crushed
- 1 shallot, sliced
- ½ red chilli, deseeded & finely chopped

- 200g/7oz tinned chopped tomatoes
- 60ml/¼ cup vegetable stock
- 1 tbsp freshly chopped basil
- Salt & pepper to taste

Method

1 Make sure the mussels are cleaned to get rid of any debris or seaweed. Place in a colander and rinse thoroughly under running water.

2 Heat the oil in a large lidded pan and gently sauté the garlic, shallots and chilli. After a few minutes increase the heat and add the chopped tomatoes and vegetable stock.

3 Place the mussels in the pan, cover with the lid and steam, for approximately 4-5 minutes, shaking the pan occasionally.

4 Tip the mussels and sauce into a shallow bowl. sprinkle with basil and serve.

CHEFS NOTE
Discard any mussels that remain shut after cooking. These should not be eaten.

MARJORAM GRILLED TUNA

295
calories per serving

Ingredients

- 1 fresh tuna steak weighing 150g/5oz
- 1 tbsp extra virgin olive oil
- 2 tsp lemon juice
- 1 tbsp freshly chopped marjoram
- 75g/3oz rocket & spinach leaves
- 75g/3oz vine ripened tomatoes, sliced
- 1 tbsp Parmesan shavings
- Lemon wedges to serve
- Salt & pepper to taste

Method

1 Preheat the grill to a medium/high heat.

2 Mix together the olive oil, lemon juice & marjoram and lightly brush on either side of the steak (reserving any remaining juice).

3 Place the tuna steak under the grill and cook for 2-3 minutes each side or until the tuna is cooked to your liking.

4 Remove from the grill, season and place on a plate with the green leaves and tomatoes. Drizzle any remaining juice over the top along with the Parmesan shavings. Serve with the lemon wedges.

CHEFS NOTE
Fresh tuna is best served rare in the centre, but feel free to adjust to your own taste.

GRILLED ASPARAGUS

220 calories per serving

Ingredients

- 125g/5oz asparagus spears
- 2 tsp olive oil
- Pinch dried chilli flakes
- 1 tsp balsamic vinegar
- 2 slices Parma ham
- Salt & pepper to taste

Method

1 Preheat the grill to a medium/high heat.

2 In a bowl mix together all the ingredients, except the ham, ensuring each asparagus spear is coated with oil. Place under the grill and cook for 4-6 minutes each side or until cooked through.

3 Remove from the grill, season and serve immediately with the Parma ham laid over the top.

CHEFS NOTE

Feel free to replace Parma ham with some finely chopped sundried tomatoes.

HALLOUMI & BULGUR WHEAT

360 calories per serving

Ingredients

- 50g/2oz sliced halloumi
- ½ onion, chopped
- ½ garlic clove, crushed
- 1 red pepper, deseeded & finely chopped

- 2 tsp olive oil
- 50g/2oz bulgar wheat
- 1 tbsp freshly chopped flat leaf parsley
- Salt & pepper to taste

Method

1 Cook the bulgur wheat in salted boiling water for 10 minutes or until tender.

2 Meanwhile gently sauté the chopped onions, garlic & peppers in the olive oil until softened.

3 In a separate pan add the halloumi . You don't need to use any oil. Cook the first side of the halloumi for a minute or two. Flip and cook for a further minutes.

4 Drain the bulgur wheat and fluff with a fork. Combine in the pan with the peppers and onions.

5 Pile into a shallow bowl. Sit the halloumi on top, sprinkle with parsley and serve.

CHEFS NOTE
This is also good with quinoa or a combination of quinoa and bulgur wheat.

FRESH HERB & TURMERIC PRAWNS

380
calories per serving

Ingredients

- 1 tsp olive oil
- 1 garlic clove, crushed
- ½ bird's-eye chilli, deseeded & finely chopped
- 200g/7oz shelled, raw king prawns
- 1 tsp turmeric
- 1 tbsp soy sauce
- 1 tbsp Thai fish sauce
- 125g/4oz wholemeal microwavable rice
- 2 tsp freshly chopped coriander/cilantro
- 2 tsp flat leaf parsley, chopped
- 1 bunch spring onions/scallions
- Salt & pepper to taste

Method

1 Heat the olive oil in a frying pan or wok and gently sauté the garlic and chillies for a minute or two.

2 Add the prawns, turmeric, soy sauce & fish sauce and cook until the prawns begin to pink up.

3 Check the prawns are cooked through, add the chopped herbs and rice to the pan. Combine for a minute or two.

4 Slice the spring onions and toss through the brown rice. Season & serve.

CHEFS NOTE
Serve with lemon wedges if you wish.

CANNELLINI BEAN SOUP

300 calories per serving

Ingredients

- 1 tbsp extra virgin olive oil
- 2 garlic cloves, peeled
- 75g/3oz celery
- 50g/2oz shallots, sliced
- 400g/14oz tinned cannellini beans
- 1.25lt/5 cups vegetable stock
- 200g/7oz whole wheat orzo pasta
- 4 tbsp pesto
- Salt & pepper to taste

Method

1 Heat the olive oil in a high-sided pan and gently sauté the garlic, celery & shallots, for a few minutes. Meanwhile cook the orzo in salted boiling water until tender, drain and put to one side.

2 Add the cannellini beans and stock to the onions, cover and leave to gently simmer for a few minutes or until tender.

3 Remove two whole ladles of cannellini beans. Blend the rest of the beans and stock to a smooth consistency, add a little boiling water if needed. Combine together the cooked orzo, smooth sauce and reserved beans and divide into shallow bowls. Dollop a serving of pesto in the middle of each bowl. Season & serve.

CHEFS NOTE
This soup serves 4 so feel free to freeze the remaining portions (leave the pesto out until serving if you are planning to freeze).

CREAMY MUSHROOM & WALNUT SPAGHETTI

450
calories per serving

Ingredients

- 25g/1oz dried porcini mushrooms
- 75g/3oz wholewheat spaghetti
- 1 tsp extra virgin olive oil
- 1 garlic clove, crushed
- 2 shallots, sliced
- 1 tsp dried thyme
- 2 tsp mascarpone cheese
- 2 tsp tomato puree/paste
- 6 walnuts halves, chopped
- 1 tbsp flat leaf parsley, chopped
- Salt & pepper to taste

Method

1 Place the porcini mushrooms in a little boiling water and leave to rehydrate for a few minutes until softened then thinly slice.

2 Cook the spaghetti in a pan of boiling water until tender.

3 Heat the olive oil in a high-sided frying pan and gently sauté the garlic, shallots & dried thyme whilst the pasta cooks.

4 When the onions are soft add the mascarpone cheese and tomato puree & stir well. Drain the cooked pasta and add to the frying pan.

5 Toss well. Season & serve with the walnuts and parsley sprinkled over the top.

CHEFS NOTE

Dried porcini mushrooms are readily available in any supermarket.

LIME CHICKEN KEBAB

470 calories per serving

Ingredients

- 50g/2oz quinoa
- 250ml/1 cup hot vegetable stock
- 1 garlic clove, crushed
- 2 tsp extra virgin olive oil
- 2 tsp lime juice
- 125g/4oz skinless chicken breast, cubed

- 50g/2oz baby spinach leaves
- 1 tbsp flat leaf parsley, chopped
- 1 tsp freshly chopped coriander/cilantro
- Salt & pepper to taste
- Metal skewers

Method

1 Put the quinoa and stock in a saucepan, cover and cook for about 10 minutes or until it's tender. (Add more stock if you need to and when it's ready drain off any excess liquid and put to one side).

2 Meanwhile preheat the grill to a medium/high heat.

3 Mix together the garlic, olive oil & lime juice in a bowl. Season the chicken and add to the bowl. Combine well and skewer each piece to make a large chicken kebab.

4 Place under the grill and cook for 6-8 minutes each side or until the chicken is cooked through and piping hot. Remove from the grill, and season.

5 Arrange the spinach and kebab on a plate, sprinkle with the chopped herbs and serve.

CHEFS NOTE
This lovely meal can be made ahead and allowed to cool for a cold lunch.

COD & OLIVES IN TOMATO SAUCE

300 calories per serving

Ingredients

- 1 tsp olive oil
- ½ red chilli, deseeded & finely sliced
- ½ onion, sliced
- 1 garlic clove, crushed
- 75g/3oz ripe plum tomatoes, roughly chopped
- 1 tbsp sundried tomato puree
- 1 tbsp pitted green olives, sliced
- 150g/5oz skinless, boneless cod fillet
- 2 tsp freshly chopped flat leaf parsley
- Salt & pepper to taste

Method

1 Gently sauté the onion, chilli and garlic in the olive oil for a few minutes until softened.

2 Add the chopped tomatoes, puree & olives and leave to gently simmer for 5 minutes stirring occasionally.

3 Season the fish fillet and cut into thick slices. Add the fish to the pan and combine well. Cover and leave to gently simmer for 8-10 minutes or until the fish is cooked through and piping hot.

4 Sprinkle with chopped parsley and serve.

CHEFS NOTE
This is even better served with a slice of fresh crusty bread to mop up all the lovely tomato juices.

JAMAICAN CHICKEN SALAD

440 calories per serving

Ingredients

- 150g/15oz skinless chicken breast
- ½ tsp crushed chilli flakes,
- 1 tbsp lime juice
- Pinch of 1 mixed spice
- 1 tsp olive oil
- ½ onion, sliced
- 2 large plum tomatoes, roughly chopped
- ½ red pepper, deseeded & sliced
- 150g/5oz mixed salad leaves
- Salt & pepper to taste

Method

1 Season the chicken and slice into thin strips.

2 Mix together the chilli flakes, lime juice, mixed spice and olive oil in a bowl to make a dressing. Add the chicken slices to the bowl and combine well.

3 Heat the oil and gently sauté the dressed chicken, onions, tomatoes and peppers in a frying pan for a few minutes (add a little more oil if needed).

4 When the chicken is cooked through arrange on a bed of mixed salad leaves to serve.

CHEFS NOTE

This dish is good served with some fat free natural yoghurt to balance the heat of chilli.

YOGA Workouts

We recommend trying to find the time to practice yoga every day. A daily session will boost physical & mental wellbeing. The three workouts which have been developed in this book can be undertaken any time of the day depending on your schedule - although you will find the Morning & Tummy Toning Yoga most suited to the day time (or when you need to be refreshed) whilst the restful sleep yoga is best suited for the very the end of the day.

The first two workouts will take around 15 minutes to complete. The third is a 30 minute relaxation session which can also be split into two 15 minute routines. All you need to get started is a mat, a block and pillows for support. That said there is no need to run out and buy any equipment at all. You can do any of these routines comfortably on a rug or carpet and the yoga block can be substituted for a small strong shoe sized box.

Yoga should never be approached as a competitive sport. It is a personal journey. Always listen to your body and never push yourself too hard. Concentrating on breathing is an extremely important part of yoga practice and you will learnt to use the rhythm of your breathing to help you move through the poses. Always move into poses on a breath exhalation and make sure you move slowly and methodically. Try to relax your facial muscles and jaw whilst tensing the muscles you should be concentrating on.

Restful Sleep Workout Tips:

When you are undertaking this workout try to concentrate on nothing other than your own breathing. Try not to alter it but instead just feel it's natural rhythm and depth. Inevitably your mind will jump around from thought to thought - seemingly uncontrollably. Try not to become frustrated by this. Instead notice where your mind is and each time gently bring your thoughts back to your breathing. This is a skill in itself and it won't come right away. Emptying your mind is not as easy as it sounds, but have patience with yourself. If you try to anchor your thoughts around your breathing and repeat this routine regularly you will learn to calm your mind and move towards a stillness which will benefit your long term well-being.

Morning YOGA

- Pose 1: **COW**
- Pose 2: **CAT**
- Pose 3: **COBRA**
- Pose 4: **EXTENSION**
- Pose 5: **ELBOW TO KNEE**
- Pose 6: **BIND**
- Pose 7: **LOW LUNGE**

- Pose 8: **LOW LUNGE STRETCH**
- Pose 9: **LIZARD POSE**
- Pose 10: **HALF SPLITS**
- Pose 11: **TWISTED MONKEY**
- Pose 12: **SIDE PLANK**
- Pose 13: **MOUNTAIN POSE**

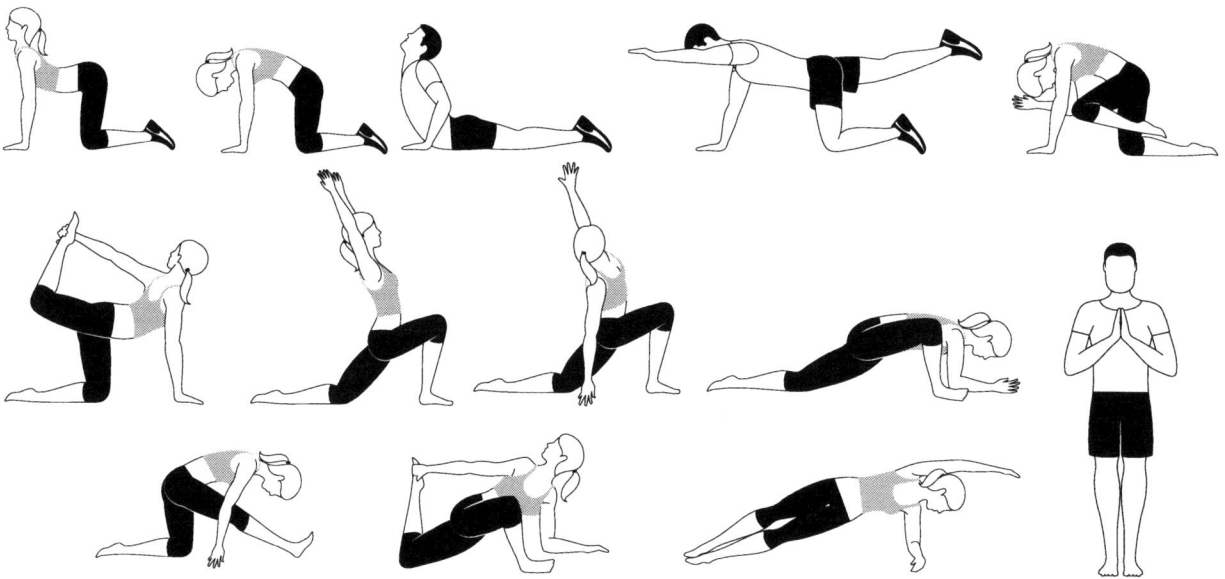

We have called this workout Morning Yoga as it is a wonderful routine to wake up with, but it can be used at any time throughout the day to refresh your mood and perk you up. It will take no more than 15 minutes and will prepare you for whatever lies ahead.

Cow

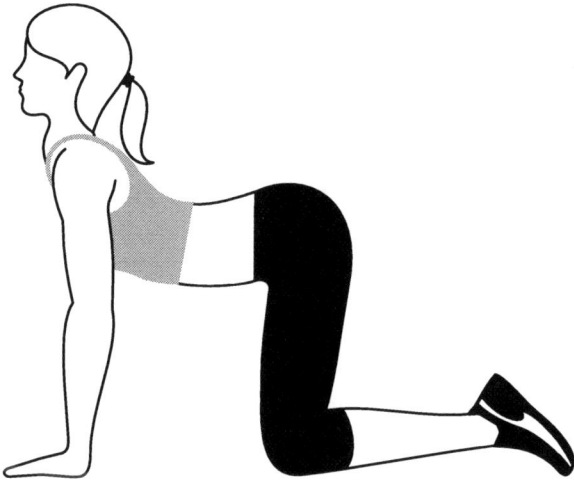

Come onto your hands and knees with hips placed over the knees. Shoulders positioned over the wrists. Your knees and hands should be shoulder distance apart, and the spine neutral. On exhalation gently lift your tail bone up to the sky, let your belly drop toward the mat and look up. Hold for a few moments before going into the next pose.

Cat

On a breath exhalation, lengthen your tail bone to the ground, draw the belly up to the spine and round the upper back like a cat. Concentrate on pressing your hands into the mat to open the shoulder blades. Let the head drop. Gently and slowly move through ten rounds of Cat/Cow, then return to a neutral spine.

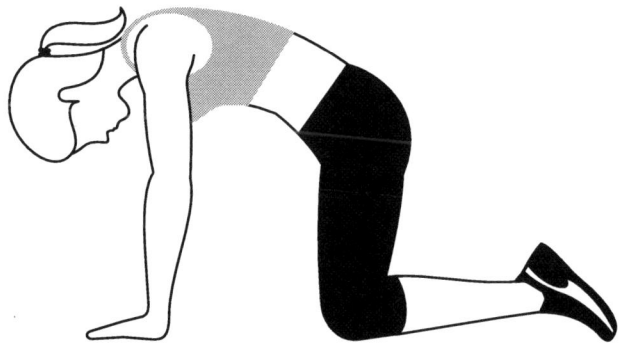

Cobra

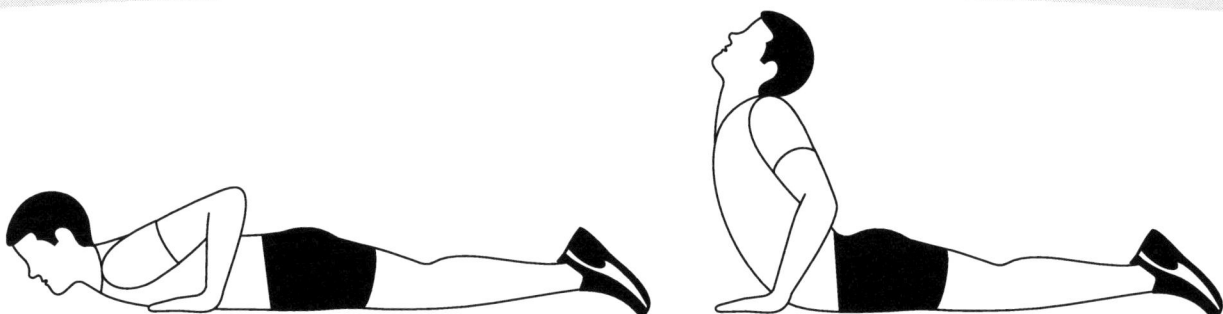

Lie face-down on mat. With elbows bent place the palms on each side of your body in line with the breastbone. Come onto fingertips and point elbows toward sky and out to sides. Press your pelvis, toes, and fingertips into the mat. On exhalation straighten the arms enough to fully lift the chest off the mat. Keep the spine long and tip the head back. Hold for 8 full deep breaths, engaging the thighs, before relaxing back onto the mat.

Extension

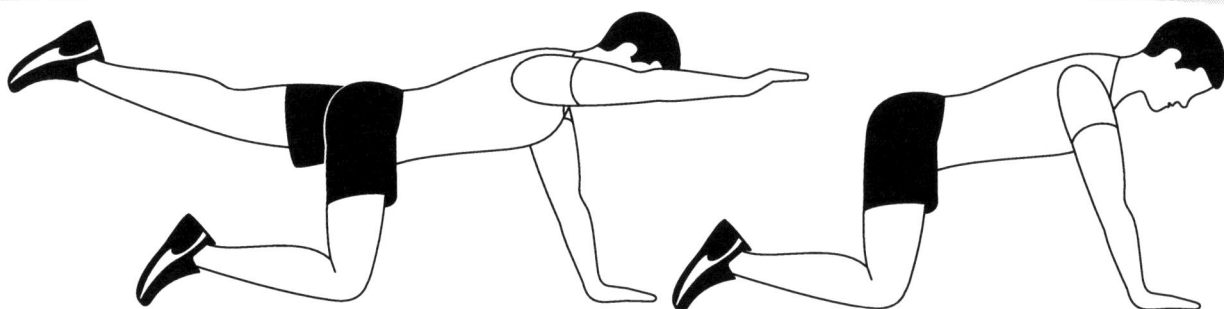

Move onto all fours. Lift your left leg and extend behind you whilst reaching your right arm forward. Lengthen your spine as you extend the arm and leg in opposite directions. Engage the core and maintain length in the back of the neck as you gaze down just in front of your hand on the mat. Hold for 5 long deep breaths. Reverse position and repeat.

Elbow To KNEE

From the extension pose move into the next pose by bringing your left elbow and your right knee in together to touch under the body. Do this on an exhalation and engage the core as you do so. Inhale to fully extend arm and leg into the extension pose and exhale to bring elbow and knee to touch. Repeat this in a careful measured way 5 times. Return to all fours ready for the next pose. Reverse position and repeat.

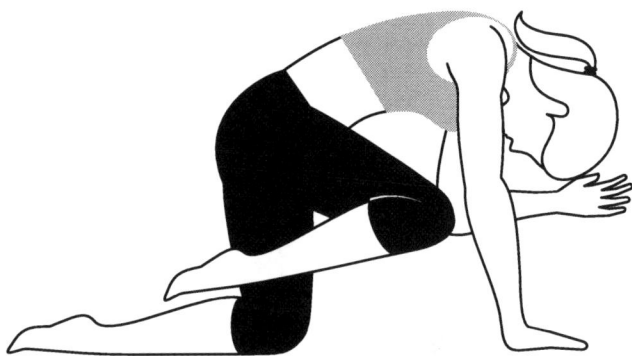

Bind

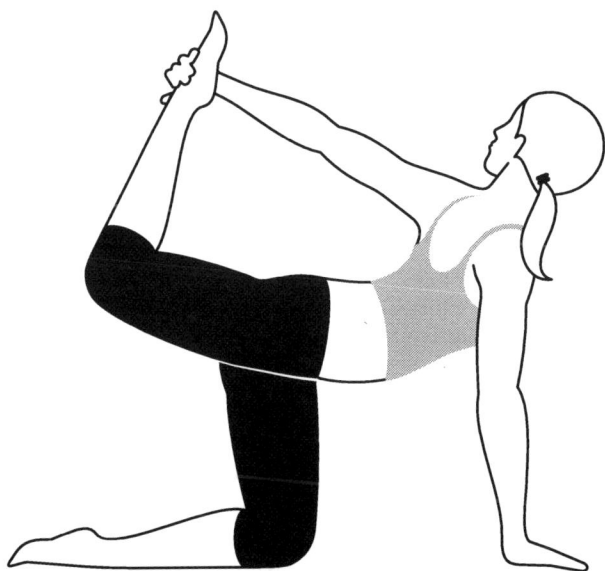

Reach left arm behind you and take hold of the right foot. Point the toes of this foot to the sky. Rolling the left shoulder toward the sky and draw the right shoulder back and down away from the right ear. Extend straight back from the hip. Hold for 5 slow deep breaths. Release from the pose. Lie on your back, hug knees to chest and gently rock side to side a few times to release the back. Reverse position and repeat.

Low LUNGE

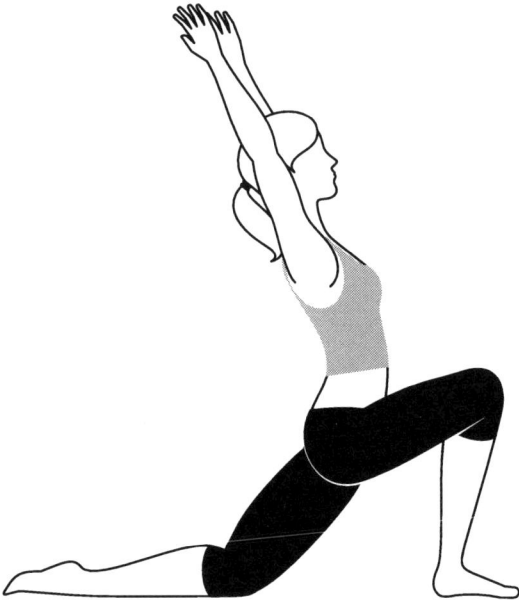

Stand straight on the mat with arms by sides. Step your right foot forward in between your hands, and on exhalation reach your arms up to the sky, keeping shoulders away from the ears. Push your right foot down and lower your hips towards the mat. Engage the core whilst avoiding puffing out the chest. Look forwards to the sky and hold the pose for 5 slow deep breaths. Reverse position and repeat.

Low Lunge STRETCH

From low lunge, reach your right fingertips down to the ground (you may wish to use a block). Exhale and reach up with the left fingertips for a full stretch. Concentrate on balance by pressing the right foot down into the mat. Look skywards but do not force your neck if this is uncomfortable. Keep the core engaged and the chest open. Feel the length of the stretch through your body and hold for 5 slow deep breaths. Reverse position and repeat.

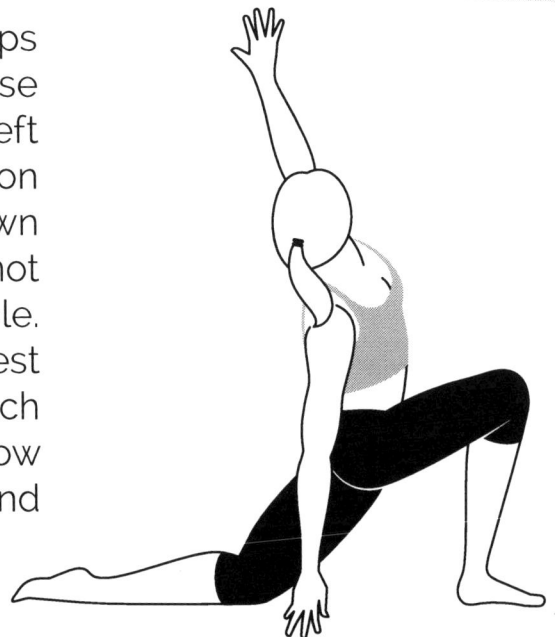

Lizard POSE

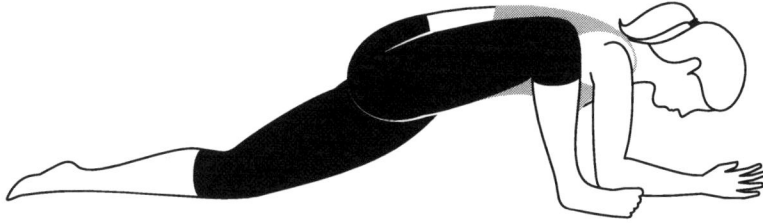

Move onto all fours on the mat. Bend the right knee and place the sole of the right foot into to the mat. On exhalation lower your body weight down to your forearms with palms facing each other. Move shoulders down away from the ears. Relax the right knee and allow it to rotate in the hip joint so that the knee falls to the right and the right foot is on its outer right edge. Do not force your knee down. Hold for 5 slow deep breaths before releasing from the pose. Reverse position and repeat.

Half SPLITS

Return to all fours. On exhalation slowly pull your hips back so that they are positioned over your left knee whilst straightening the right leg. Press your right heel into the mat, lengthen the right leg and flex the toes of the right foot back towards you. Keep the neck straight and look to the floor. Engage the core and hold for 5 slow deep breaths. Reverse position and repeat.

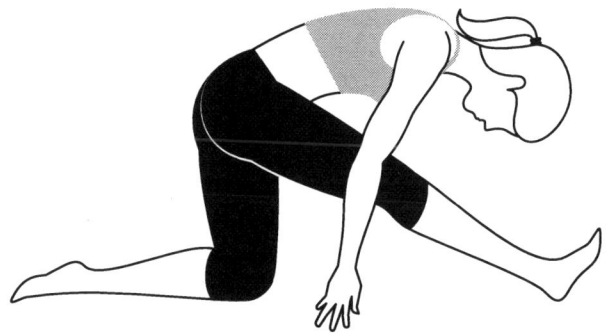

Twisted MONKEY

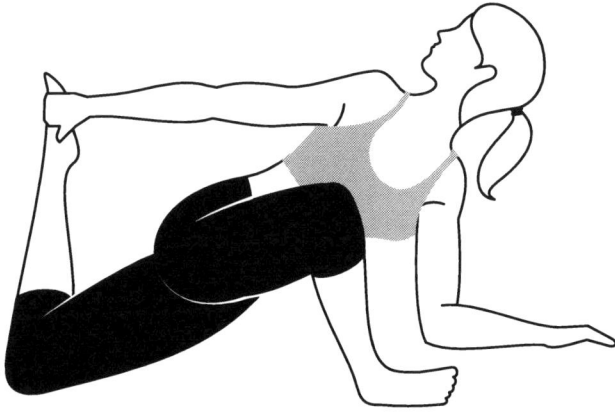

Return to all fours. On exhalation reach the right arm up and then back to take hold of your left foot. Roll the right shoulder back opening the chest. The left forearm should be flat on the mat with the palm extended. Allow the right knee to gently drop towards the floor as you come onto the outer edge of your right foot. Carefully lean the upper body back and hold for 5 slow deep breaths. Reverse position and repeat.

Side PLANK

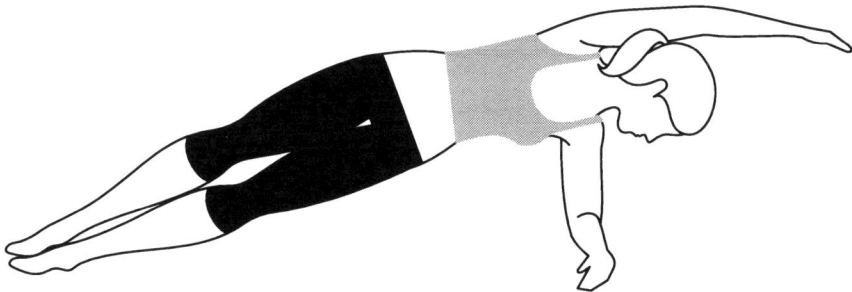

From Twisted Monkey moving your left forearm parallel to the top of the mat. Straighten the legs so that they rest on top of each other. Engage the core, extend the left arm over your head and lift the weight of your body to move into the side plank position. Feel the stretch through the side body and hold for 5 slow deep breaths. If you need stability split your legs so that both feet touch the floor. Reverse position and repeat.

Mountain POSE

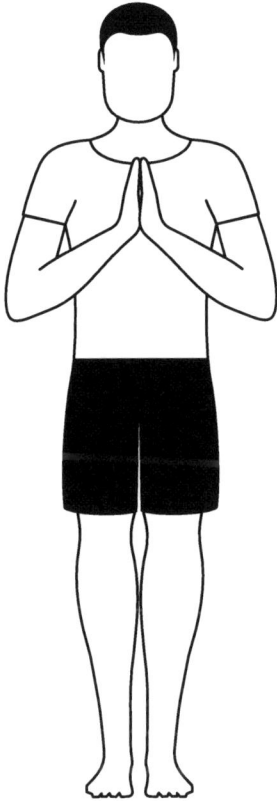

Finish the session with Mountain Pose by standing straight with legs and feet together, heels slightly apart, and arms at sides with palms facing forward. Keep your spine long, shoulders rolled back and away from the ears, spread the toes and press soles of the feet into mat. Engage thighs and lower belly, bring the gaze of the eyes towards the floor some distance ahead of you and lightly close the eyes. Slowly bring hands together at the centre of the chest and hold for 10 long deep breaths.

Tummy Toning YOGA

- Pose 1: **MOUNTAIN POSE**
- Pose 2: **STANDING LEAN**
- Pose 3: **COBRA**
- Pose 4: **MOUNTAIN CHAIR**
- Pose 5: **WARRIOR POSE**

- Pose 6: **CHEST OPENER**
- Pose 7: **DOWNWARD DOG**
- Pose 8: **PARTIAL PLANK**
- Pose 9: **PARTIAL SIDE PLANK**

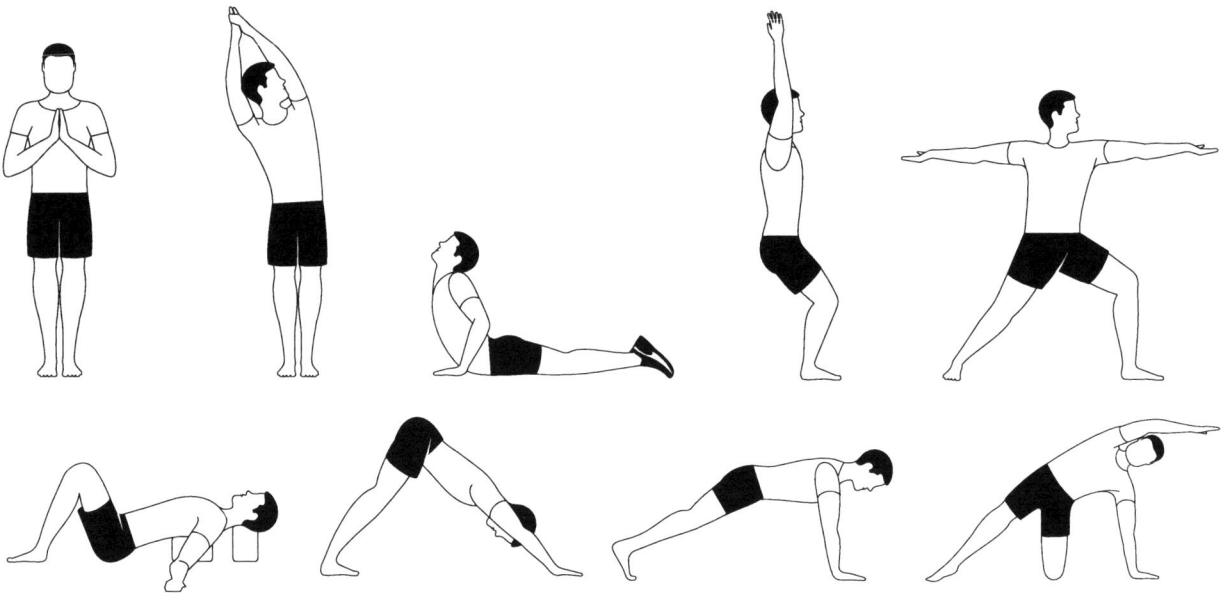

This routine is ideal for helping to tighten your core and it's also good for the thighs. Each of the poses will encourage you to use many of the core muscles we often forget about and should take no more than 15 minutes.

Mountain POSE

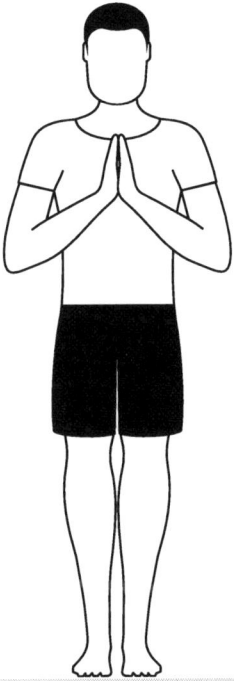

Begin the session with this iconic yoga pose by standing straight with legs and feet together, heels slightly apart, and arms at sides with palms facing forward. Keep your spine long, shoulders rolled back and away from the ears, spread the toes and press soles of the feet into mat. Engage thighs and core, bring the gaze of the eyes towards the floor some distance ahead of you and lightly close the eyes. Slowly bring hands together at the centre of the chest and hold for 10 long deep breaths.

Standing LEAN

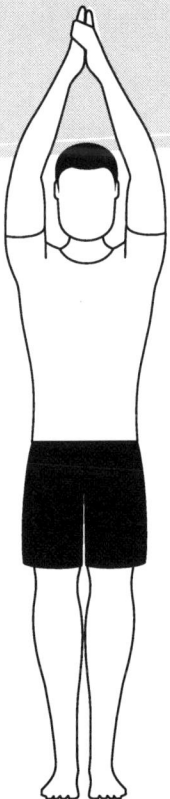

Begin by gently joining the palms above the head with the arms straight. Squeeze the inner arms in toward the ears but keep the shoulders down away from the ears. On your breath exhalation, press feet down, engage thighs and core, and stretch up and evenly over to right. Repeat the pose this time on the left side. Remember to engage the core and thighs each time and move on exhalation. Do this slowly on each side 4 times.

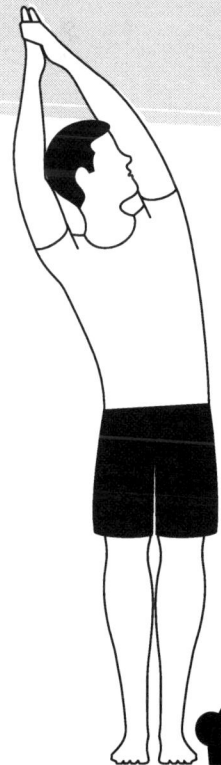

Cobra

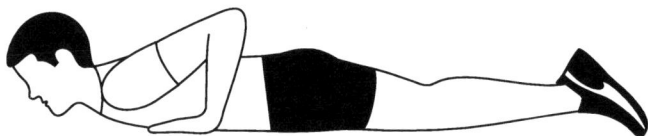

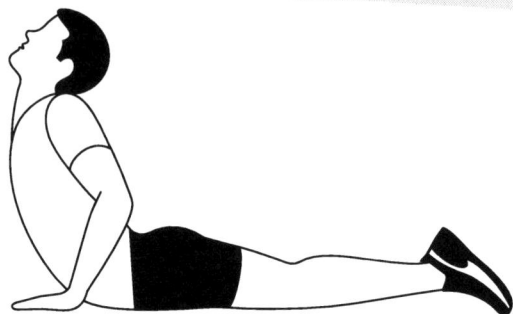

Lie face-down on mat. With elbows bent place the palms on each side of your body in line with the breastbone. Come onto fingertips and point elbows toward sky and out to sides. Press your pelvis, toes, and fingertips into the mat. On exhalation straighten the arms enough to fully lift the chest off the mat. Keep the spine long and tip the head back. Hold for 8 full deep breaths, engaging the core & thighs, before relaxing back onto the mat.

Mountain CHAIR

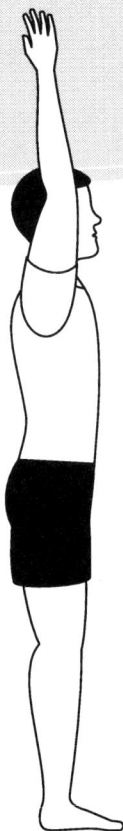

Stand straight with arms above the head and palms facing each other. On exhalation, sweep arms down and behind your body, bending knees and lowering hips. Inhale and reach arms overhead, biceps by ears with palms turned in toward each other, and sit into chair pose strongly engaging the core. On your next exhalation return to start. Repeat 10 times in a slow measured way.

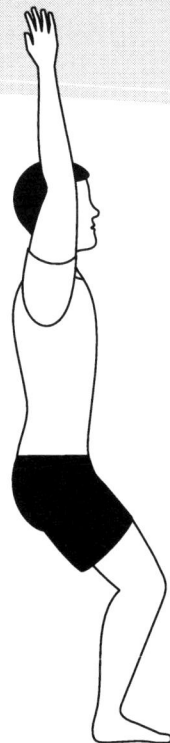

Warrior POSE

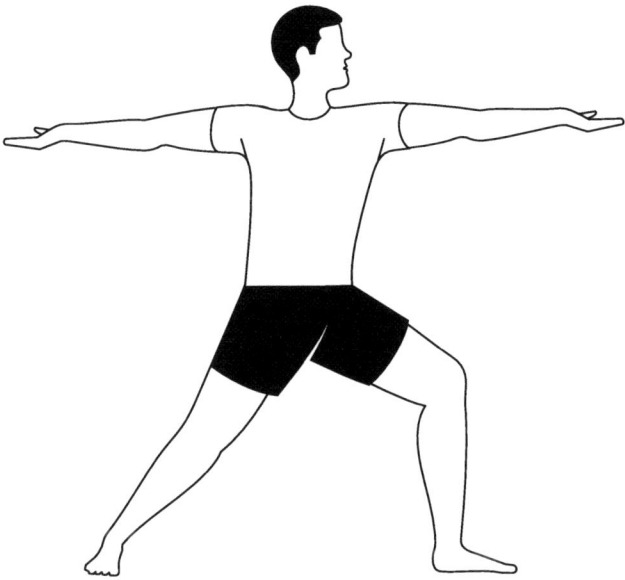

Extend the arms out at shoulder height and step your feet apart so they are positioned below the extended wrists. Have the outer edge of back foot parallel to back of mat and toes of front foot pointing forward. Engage the core and slowly bend front knee, lining it up over front ankle, and come into warrior pose with palms up.

On exhalation, straighten your front leg and sweep the arms overhead, bringing palms together . On inhalation, return to warrior pose. Repeat 8 times. Switch legs and repeat.

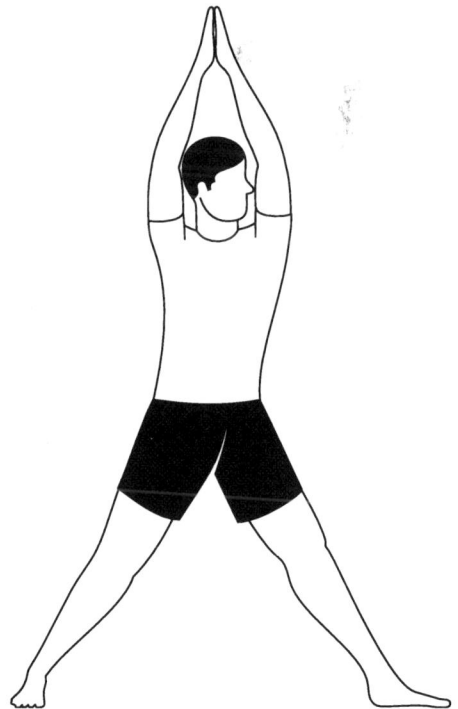

Chest OPENER

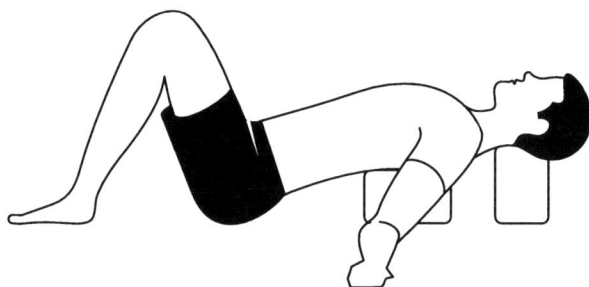

Lie face-up on mat with knees bent and feet positioned hip-width apart. Place a yoga block beneath your head and another lengthwise between shoulder blades. Bring arms out to sides and allow your chest to open. Engage your core strongly. Breathe through your stretch and stay in this pose for 2 minutes.

Downward DOG

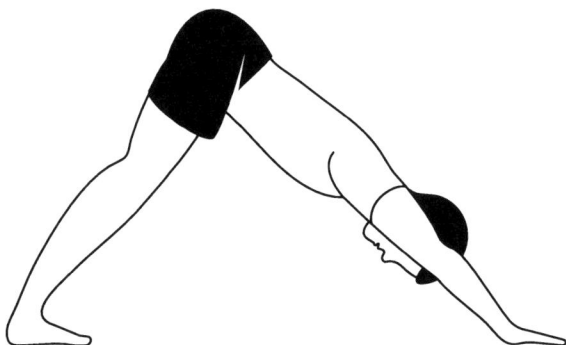

Start on all fours with knees and hands hip-width apart . Curl the feet to push toes into mat. On exhalation push down into hands and feet. Engage the core strongly and lift hips to sky keeping the back straight as if you are trying to push the mat away from yourself with your hands. Press down strongly through arms and balls of feet and lower heels onto the mat (don't worry if you have to bend your knees a little). Hold for 5 deep breaths keeping the core and thighs engaged throughout.

Partial PLANK

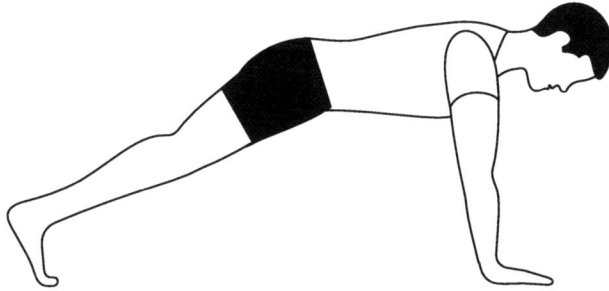

From Downward Dog, exhale and bring your body forward to come into the pose. Lengthen your spine and press heels towards the back of the room, engaging your core and thighs. Hold this position for a few moments then on exhalation, push down back into the downward dog pose. Keep the core and thighs engaged as you repeat this slowly 7 times.

Partial Side PLANK

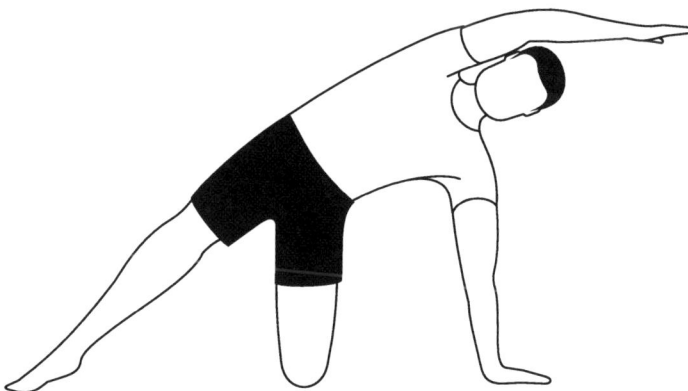

Move onto your knees. Extend the right leg whilst the left stays rooted to the floor. On exhalation turn your body to the right, shifting your weight onto left palm and right foot. Keep your spine and neck in line as you extend the right arm overhead, with palm facing down. Hold for 8 full deep breaths. Repeat on opposite side.

Restful Sleep YOGA

- Pose 1: **COW**
- Pose 2: **CAT**
- Pose 3: **BRIDGE POSE**
- Pose 4: **LEGS UP THE WALL**
- Pose 5: **SEATED FORWARD BEND**
- Pose 6: **WIDE LEG FORWARD BEND**
- Pose 7: **COBRA**
- Pose 8: **LEFT NOSTRIL BREATHING**

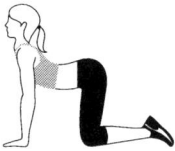

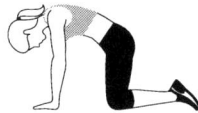

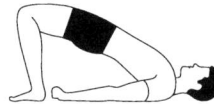

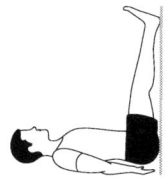

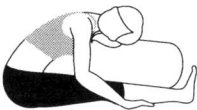

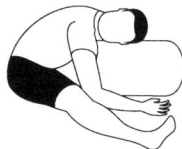

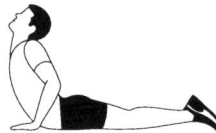

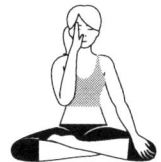

This gentle routine is ideal for preparing for bed, winding down in the evening or if you wish to meditate/rest throughout the day. You will need to have a mat and some pillows to hand and it should take no more than 30 minutes. You can split this session into two 15 minutes routines if this works better for you. Feel free to lengthen or shorten each of the poses to suit your own schedule.

Cow

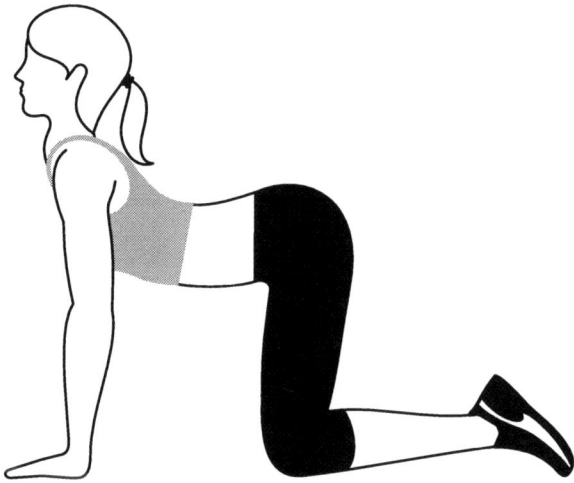

Come onto your hands and knees with hips placed over the knees. Shoulders positioned over the wrists. Your knees and hands should be shoulder distance apart, and the spine neutral. On exhalation gently lift your tail bone up to the sky, let your belly drop toward the mat and look up. Hold for a few moments before going into the next pose.

Cat

On a breath exhalation, lengthen your tail bone to the ground, draw the belly up to the spine and round the upper back like a cat. Concentrate on pressing your hands into the mat to open the shoulder blades. Let the head drop. Gently and slowly move through ten rounds of Cat/Cow, then return to a neutral spine.

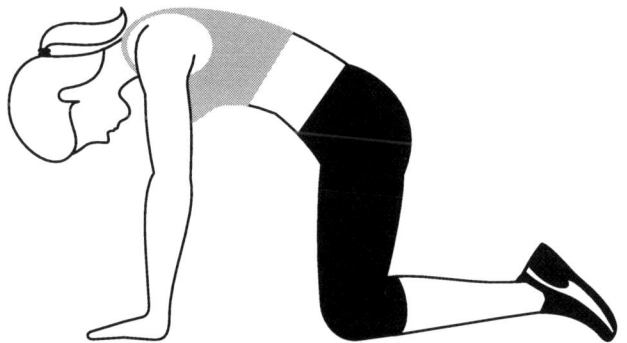

Bridge POSE

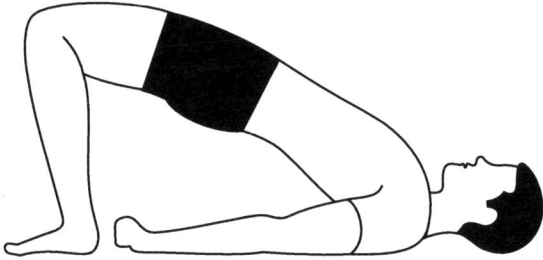

On your mat lie down with feet flat on the floor hip-width apart. Place your hands beside you with palms facing down. Engage your thighs and core and on exhalation lift your body up so that your back is flat and your knees are at a 45 degree angle whilst your arms remain flat on the floor. Settle into the pose and hold it for 2-3 minutes if you can.

Legs Up THE WALL

Position yourself on your mat side-on close up to wall. Roll onto your back with your legs up in the air. Twist yourself around 90 degrees so that your legs rest straight up against the wall. Shuffle your bottom up tight against the wall if you need to. Keep your arms straight by your side with the palms flat down. Remain in this pose for 5 minutes breathing deeply and slowly, concentrating on nothing other than movement and feeling of your breath.

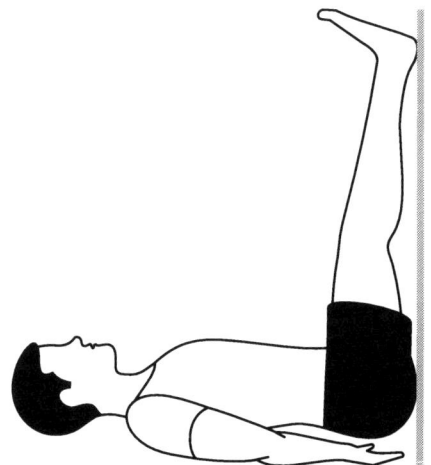

Seated Forward BEND

Sit on the mat with your legs straight out in front of you. Place pillow(s) on your thighs against your stomach (you may need to experiment with the height of the support). Put your arms above your head then reach forward as you bend your body onto the pillow and rest the side of your head onto the pillow support. Allow your arms to rest by your side and remain in this position for 5 minutes.

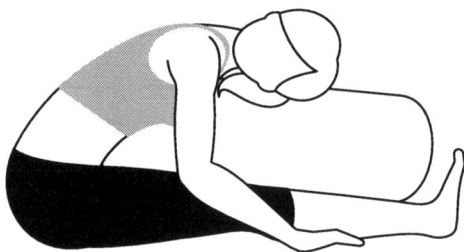

Wide Leg Forward BEND

This is a variation on the last pose. This time move your legs apart whilst you are in an upright sitting position. Place your cushion(s) onto the floor between your legs. Put your arms above your head then reach forward as you bend your body onto the pillow and rest the side of your head onto the pillow support – use the opposite side of your head from the last pose. Allow your arms to rest by your side and remain in this position for 5 minutes. If this feels uncomfortable it can be helpful to sit on a block or cushion to lift your pelvis or/and you may wish to bend your knees a little.

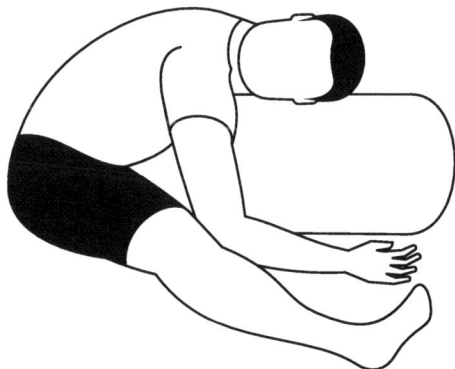

Cobra

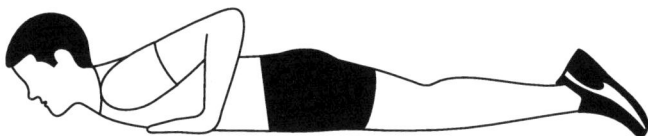

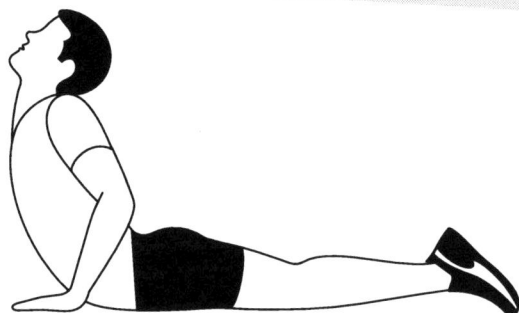

Lie face-down on mat. With elbows bent place palms a little away from each side of your body in line with the breastbone. Come onto fingertips and point elbows toward sky and out to sides Press pelvis, toes, and fingertips into floor. On exhalation straighten the arms enough to lift the chest off the mat. Keep the spine long and tip the head back. Hold for 8 full deep breaths before relaxing back onto the mat.

Left Nostril BREATHING

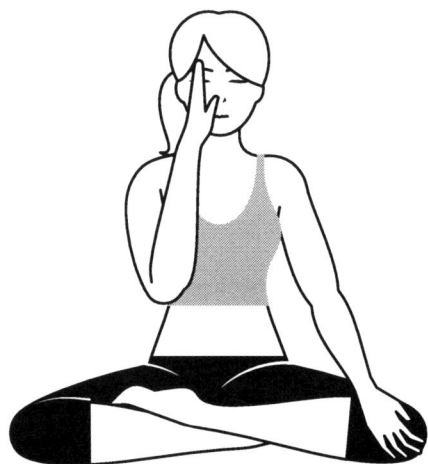

Sit in a comfortable cross- legged position. Keep your back straight with your shoulders low down away from your ears. Try to imagine a piece of string being pulled from above lifting the crown of your head up towards the sky. Cover your right nostril with your thumb or finger and begin breathing in and out through your left nostril. Breathe like this for at least 2 minutes.

This may seem strange but breathing through the left nostril has a calming effect on the nervous system and aids mediation and restful sleep.

Other COOKNATION TITLES

If you enjoyed **The** *Skinny* **15 Minute Meals & Yoga Workout Plan** you may also be interested in other *Skinny* titles in the CookNation series.

Visit **www.bellmackenzie.com** to browse the full catalogue.

Manufactured by Amazon.ca
Bolton, ON